KEEP MOVING

KEEP MOVING

Lessons on Staying Young in Mind and Body from India's Fittest Family

Milind Soman,
Ankita Konwar and
Usha Soman

with

Roopa Pai

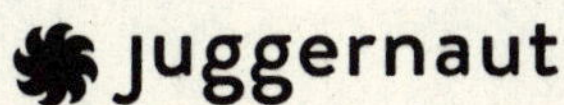

JUGGERNAUT BOOKS
C-I-128, First Floor, Sangam Vihar, Near Holi Chowk,
New Delhi 110080, India

First published by Juggernaut Books 2024

10 9 8 7 6 5 4 3 2 1

P-ISBN: 9789353457297
E-ISBN: 9789353459925

Typeset in Brandon Grotesque by R. Ajith Kumar, Noida

Printed at Replika Press Pvt. Ltd.

CONTENTS

INTRODUCTION

How do you count your age? In years and experience, and the wisdom they are supposed to bestow upon you, or by your body's strength, stamina and agility? Does youthfulness have more to do with how you feel in your head – how curious, how fresh, how hopeful, how engaged with the world and its wonders – than how many times you have circumambulated the sun? Does old age come to us, whether we are 17 or 70, when we realize that we are unable to do as much physically as those we share our birth years with? Is good health a credible marker of youth?

Which begs the obvious question: what is good health, anyway? Where does fitness, that much-bandied-about word, erm, *fit* into this picture? Which is a subset of which?

This book sets out to find some answers to these and other important questions about age, health and well-being by exploring these themes with three remarkable individuals separated in age by over half a century, all of them part of what is arguably India's first family of fitness.

The age-defying Usha Soman, who became a social media sensation at 77 when a video of her running barefoot on a highway in a saree alongside her famous son went viral, is 84. Her son, Milind Soman, now 58, was a teenage national swimming champion who came to running at 37 and went on to wow the country with the endurance challenges he took on and completed, including, when he was 51, the gruelling Ultraman Triathlon. Milind's wife, Ankita Konwar, whose life was rocked by devastating personal tragedy, depression and addiction in her twenties, fought her way into the light, chose fitness and now matches her husband step for step, whether it is summiting Mount Kilimanjaro or completing the Mumbai marathon. As a qualified yoga teacher and practitioner, she has also moved out of his shadow into her own sphere.

These three individuals have, at first glance, very different lifestyles, fitness regimens and food habits. They also grew up very differently from each other. Born in pre-Independence India, Usha had never heard of 'exercise' as a concept. As a young man, Milind rode the wave of India's economic liberalization in the '90s and became the country's top male supermodel, kicking back into the louche alcohol–nicotine–substance lifestyle that came with the territory for over a decade. As for Ankita, she spent much of her noughties childhood in a boarding school in small-town Assam, where she thought very little about fitness or sport, dreaming instead of finding a job that would let her travel the world.

And yet, despite traversing such disparate routes, the three are now at the same summit, the one we all wish we could scale – peak fitness at their respective ages.

What does fitness look like from the perches of 84, 58, 32? What insights into the nature of health and well-being have each of them garnered along the way? What advice can they give the rest of us who admire and want to emulate them? Dozens of in-person interviews, WhatsApp questions, voice notes and phone calls later, straightforward, even commonsensical, lessons, based on a remarkably similar philosophy, emerged. Here they are.

1. Fitness and health are subsets of a larger and more holistic concept – well-being. It encompasses physical, mental and emotional health, none of which can exist without the others. You have to work on each of them consistently – no cheat days!
2. It is never too late to begin the journey to physical fitness, but embarking on it early gives you a head start. If you enjoyed an active childhood and good nutrition, thanks to opportunity, environment and encouragement – lucky you! – you are already halfway there.
3. We all lose ourselves a little as we grapple with all the stuff life tosses at us; the challenge lies in pulling

ourselves back from the brink, asking ourselves what well-being truly means to us, and pursuing it single-mindedly. Health goals! Fitness goals! Less-life-drama goals!

4. Getting back on course is difficult, but staying the course is harder. To set time aside, day after day, to move, lift, stretch and centre yourself, no matter what the demands of the world, will feel like a chore. Do it! The rewards are inestimable.
5. There is no magic-bullet diet, no miracle regimen, to peak fitness. All learning, understanding and wisdom of what food and activity works best for each of us can only be figured out by . . . each of us! Bummer!
6. However clichéd it may sound, age IS just a number. The body changes with age, there's no help for that, but if you listen to your body closely and tweak your diet and exercise based on what it is telling you, you will enjoy good health at every age.
7. Let go of negativity, don't be judgemental, practise gratitude, open yourself to new and uncomfortable experiences, be kind to yourself, accept the things you cannot change without bitterness. Ta-da! You have brewed the other secret sauce to wellness!
8. It is spectacularly unintelligent not to make our health and well-being our No. 1 priority. Our survival, our very

existence, depends on it. Why in heaven's name haven't you done it yet?

9. The trick, if there is such a thing, is to keep moving – moving on from past regret, moving forward towards the next adventure, moving old ideas along to accommodate new ones, moving your goalposts, moving your limbs. Fight lazy, keep moving!

Out the door yet to beat your own path to peak fitness? Hang on a minute. Maybe it's best to read the book before you go, for as Usha, Milind and Ankita tell us, they arrived at these secrets to well-being over years and years of experimenting, experiencing, rising, falling and picking themselves up again. No shortcuts, remember?

And that's why this book is as much a memoir as a self-help book or a meditation on the nature of fitness and health. Walk beside the Somans on the paths they travelled by, seeing their very different journeys through their own eyes, hearing their stories, often extraordinary in their ordinariness, watching them role-model 'best health' practices for the rest of us. In doing so, you will be inspired to become, and remain, like them, ageless.

WHAT DOES FITNESS LOOK LIKE AT 84?

'In your seventies and eighties, your body is most certainly in decline. Your metabolism slows, making digestion difficult. Balance becomes a problem. Your joints begin to wear down palpably. You may slowly begin to lose faculties like hearing and short-term memory. At this stage, adapt your activities to the changing state of your body, but don't stop moving. Include a low-impact exercise routine like age-appropriate yoga, stretches and swimming to keep the joints lubricated and improve mobility. Walk as much as you comfortably can. Cut out heavy foods like red meat from your diet. Eat fewer meals a day. As for the mind, don't allow it to dwell in the past. Don't let anyone tell you that you cannot do something because of your age. People around you, especially your children, mean well when they tell you to slow down, but they don't know what you're capable of. Why, YOU don't know what you are capable of! Stay positive, stay cheerful, stay curious and set yourself new challenges – and you may end up surprising yourself, as I did.' – **Usha**

WHAT DOES FITNESS LOOK LIKE AT 58?

'60 may be the new 40 according to lifestyle magazines, but Nature has her own rules. You are at your prime between the

ages of 20 and 30, ripe for procreation, which is the only thing Nature cares about. After 30, both body and mind go into slow, imperceptible decline. The most we can do is to try and arrest that decline. At 58, what becomes important is efficiency – you may not have as much energy as you did before, so you must use what you have in the most optimal way. One way to do that is to identify weaknesses and work on those instead of trying to do everything. As you age, for instance, you begin to feel the effects of gravity – counter them by moving your body against gravity, with pull-ups, squats, headstands. Adaptability takes a hit – you are no longer as agile in body and mind. It takes longer to acquire new skills, cope with changing technology and recover from injuries and setbacks. Push yourself every day but in a way that is comfortable. Let go of the ego, focus on being at peace, and make the experience and wisdom of your years work for you.' – **Milind**

WHAT DOES FITNESS LOOK LIKE AT 32?

'In your twenties and early thirties, your body is in its prime – all you need to do to keep it functioning at its optimum capacity is a little maintenance from time to time. But your mind – ah, that's quite another matter. At this stage of life, the mind is most fragile and vulnerable and needs your full

attention and nurturing. Make building a strong, empowered mind – often accomplished through an active body – your primary responsibility. Everything else will flow from there.'
– **Ankita**

SECTION 1

STARTING STRONG

The Launch Sets the Course

How much of 'good health' is nature, hardwired into our genes? What fraction of a strong body and mind do we owe to nurture, especially in terms of what we grow up eating and what habits and disciplines are inculcated into us in childhood? How significantly can each of us, by thoughtfully and assiduously cultivating ways of being and living in adulthood, fashion the course of our health destinies? The jury is out, and will probably always be, on the exact proportions of these three determining factors, but one thing is for sure – a good, solid start is a treasure not to be scoffed at.

USHA

My Bombay Childhood

'Exercise? My generation had never heard of the concept. Stretches, bends, lifts, squats – they were all part of daily routine. Exercise had to be invented for the generation that came after, newly freed from physical labour.'

I had just turned eight when India became independent – I'll leave it to you to figure out the year of my birth. My parents traced their family roots to Goa, but my five siblings – an older sister, two younger sisters and two younger brothers – and I had a proper Bombay childhood.

I suppose our household of ten was a little unusual by today's standards. There was my father, a well-respected doctor. There was my mother, who had had very little formal education, and would go on to birth six children – in two lots, as it were. Kumud, Pushpa and I were born between 1935 and 1940, with me in the middle, and Vinayak, Surendra and Kalpana came after an eleven-year gap, between 1951 and 1954. There was my mother's young sister, our aunt, just eight years older than Kumud. My father had sent for her from my mother's ancestral village, so that she could attend school with us in Bombay and be educated. That accounts for nine people.

The tenth, and we come now to the unusual part, was my father's second wife, much younger than my own mother. This was before the Hindu Marriage Act of 1955 was enacted, so there was nothing illegal about it, but thinking back on it now, I'm surprised that my mother didn't feel – or at least never showed – any resentment towards her, especially considering the way in which she entered our family.

When World War II broke out in 1939, people did not at first realize how much displacement it would cause of people and materials over the next six years. Bombay emptied out, and doctors were among the first professionals to be dispatched to remote locations. At some point during the war, my father was sent off to Goa. He returned just after the war ended, with a young woman doctor in tow. I was only six or seven then, so I don't remember how exactly he broke the news to my mother, but from that day on, we had a stepmother.

I cannot say that my mother and stepmother were friends, but there was absolutely no discord between them. There was a clear division of responsibilities – the younger stepped out each morning with my father, to work alongside him at his dispensary; the older took care of the house and the children. Kumud, Pushpa and I, along with my aunt, helped my mother with the domestic work in the day, and read and swapped books with my stepmother when she returned from work, enjoying the discussions that followed. It was all very pleasant and harmonious. Things might have been different if my stepmother had had children of her own, but much as she wanted them, it never came to pass. I daresay that it was we children who benefited most from the situation.

We were a well-to-do family, and ours was a happy, comfortable childhood, with lots of friends in the neighbourhood. My father never restricted his daughters in play – in an age when it was unusual to see girls on bicycles, the three of us spent our weekends cycling down the leafy lanes around our home with abandon. We were first sent to a girls' school and then to a co-ed one, where we participated in all kinds of sports and athletic activities – running, three-legged races, langda (you hopped on one foot to 'catch' the others, who were running circles around you), kho-kho, hu-tu-tu (or kabaddi – very popular when I was young and very popular again these days). We didn't play volleyball or throwball in those days – those were 'foreign' games.

Oh, there was also skipping rope! I was very good at it, quite the champ. My talent in this department came into full flow during Ganesh Utsav, at the skipping competitions held in the pandal near our home – the last one standing, or in this case, skipping, won the prize, and that girl was usually me. I could go up to 500 skips without a pause at those contests!

In my time, as I remember it, everyone was active, even in a city. Owning a car, or even a scooter – in fact, scooters came well after cars – was not a common thing, so people simply walked from place to place. Plus, there were no gadgets to lighten your load, whether it was housework or anything else. If you are doing all the housework yourself, where is the need for a gym? The word exercise was unheard of – it was only wrestlers and bodybuilders and serious sportspeople who, to use a phrase from today, 'worked out'. There was never any mention of yoga either, leave alone an International Yoga Day.

I have always been blessed with good health – I was seldom ill as a child. I rarely even felt out of sorts, because of, say, a change in weather, like other children did. I don't remember my parents being unwell either, or having any kind of predisposition to respiratory or digestive conditions. My little brother Surendra contracted polio as a child of seven or eight – remember this was a time before American virologist Jonas Salk developed the first effective polio vaccine in 1952 – and was treated with ayurvedic oil massages. To everyone's delight – but not their surprise, for everyone trusted the treatment implicitly – he recovered completely.

Surendra went on to become a surgeon in the UK. He has only just retired. My older sister Kumud lives in Goa and continues to have an active life. Pushpa is a lawyer – she represented BEST (Brihanmumbai Electric Supply and Transport) and MMRDA (Mumbai Metropolitan Region Development Authority) in her day, and still goes to court for them on occasion. I myself was very keen to be a doctor, but did not manage to secure the marks needed for admission. I studied biochemistry instead. As for the others, Vinayak became a civil engineer, and the youngest, Kalpana, is an occupational therapist.

'The healthy food "rules" that everyone proclaims these days as if they were brand-new scientific discoveries – Eat fresh! Eat local! Eat seasonal! – were simply part of our lives. Eating healthy was our default mode because there was no store-bought "junk food" to be had.'

This may be an anecdotal memory, but it seems to me that there were fewer diseases then. Or maybe they hadn't been named yet. The BCG (Bacillus Calmette-Guerin) vaccine was already available, as was the smallpox vaccine, so children were protected to that extent. Typhoid was rare, cholera absent in the city. Even influenza wasn't common.

Maybe that was because everyone followed some time-honoured traditional practices, like washing their hands and feet before they entered the house. Maybe it was because no one ate out, and there was really no 'fast food' or 'junk food' to be had.

In our home, as in other middle-class homes like ours, my mother cooked for the family. We enjoyed our vegetables, along with chicken and mutton, except on Mondays and Saturdays, which were meat-free. My mother, as I have already mentioned, was from Goa, so there was a lot of fish (five times a week, on average) and a lot of coconut in our food. We ate more rice than chapati when we were young – chapati was added on slowly as we grew up. We had no refrigerator, of course, so every meal was cooked fresh. I do think the quality of fruits and vegetables was better in those days, and we only ate seasonal vegetables and fruits. The kind of obsessive conversations around food that happen these days, and the 'rules' that are routinely dished out as if they were brand-new scientific discoveries – Eat fresh! Eat local! Eat seasonal! – were simply part of our lives. These food practices were so universal – and so commonsensical – that no one found the need to talk about them.

Families were large in themselves, and many lived under the same roof as the extended family, in the joint-family system. People met each other a lot more, casually, not just for work or on special occasions. We visited people often, dropped in when we felt like seeing friends and relatives – there was never any need to 'plan' a visit. Even though there were very few telephones, leave alone smartphones and social media, we knew what was happening in people's lives, and were there to support each other in times of joy and grief. If someone was ill, a relative would come to stay for as long as she was needed, and take over the cooking and the children. Mattresses would be rolled out on the floor, and overnight visitors would be accommodated without a second thought in tiny homes – people shared space, food and time generously with each other.

These days, people's lives are so overscheduled that there is no room for impromptu meetings – my sister and I, even though we live in the same city, do not meet for months on end because of the planning involved in making it happen. Wishing people 'Happy Birthday' on WhatsApp may feel like a connection to young people today, but it doesn't to me. I would say that we were certainly a lot more 'connected' when I was growing up – with our families, our neighbours and the larger community – than we are now. Those connections may also have been a factor in promoting good health, especially mental health.

It is robust mental health that helps one deal with difficult life situations, and that is helped along by making deep human connections. When you interact with other people closely, as a young person – spending time at their homes, eating their food, observing how other families interact with each other – you understand that although people are different, that doesn't make them or their way of life superior or inferior to yours. You become less judgemental of other people's choices and motivations; you simply accept them. That kind of acceptance of differences, in itself, goes a long way towards lightening one's mind, for most of our stress is caused by our inability to embrace people and situations for what they are.

'Eating dinner together every day is a great family bonding exercise for sure, but what makes it vital is that it allows parents to observe their children closely, and become aware of small changes in mood and behaviour.'

I have not lived the life of a young parent in the twenty-first century, and I am sure they are trying their best, but it seems to me that what I understood as parenting doesn't exist anymore.

It was different in our time. Children had fewer distractions, and were around the house a lot, which made it easier to manage them. Parents had fewer distractions, so there was more opportunity to observe the children and catch subtle shifts in behaviour and mood. The shared evening meal was a daily bonding exercise – with 'eating out' not an option, family members had no choice but to be present at dinnertime. Conversation was easy and casual, rarely about logistics and scheduling. Even the youngest child had some awareness of what was going on in everyone else's life, because it was all shared during the meal.

Today, people living under the same roof seldom eat a meal together at home in a relaxed manner, discussing their day. Significantly more worrisome, children rarely have a childhood. Sure, they know a lot – I would say too much! – more than their parents did at that age, but all that 'knowledge' leads inevitably to a loss of mental and emotional innocence. When you know and have too much too soon, the natural fallout is boredom. That is why everyone is constantly seeking something new – a new gadget, a new kind of food, a new experience. The real problem is that while children have the knowledge of things, they have no idea *how* to use that knowledge, *what* to do with it, or *in what ways* it may affect them.

Parents are always saying they have no time, but I often wonder if the truth lies in the disruption of the routine that used to rule our lives. There is so much choice now, in terms of what one can eat and where one can go and what one can do with one's time, and that choice can be exercised without too much planning. On a whim, you can have food delivered, call a cab, book tickets for a movie – why wouldn't you do it when it's all so easy, so convenient, so *exciting*? More importantly, it is what makes the kids happy! But that kind of unpredictable lifestyle also leaves the mind fragmented and anxious. No wonder so many parents feel so helpless and overstretched all the time. The thing is, being truly present for children involves the kind of immersion and calm that is not easy to summon up when you are simultaneously checking your phone for updates on pizza delivery, or being badgered by the cab driver for directions.

What a lot of young parents do have today is more money than parents did in the past, and in their keenness to compensate for the lack of quiet, involved time with their children, they spend money on them instead. Very often, they give money to the children themselves, as pocket money, to spend as they wish. That, in my opinion, is ill-advised, unless you balance the independence and freedom – both wonderful things – that you are offering your child with appropriate amounts of responsibility and accountability. One without the other is a recipe for disaster, but in my limited observation, I find that this is what often happens.

Life is significantly simpler, and temptations more easily warded off, when you are only ever given enough money to cover the bus ride to school.

MILIND

My British-Indian Childhood

'I was always the misfit – in England, I was the strange brown boy in kindergarten; in my Mumbai school, I was bullied for being too "posh". It taught me a lesson for life: how people saw me was more about who they were than who I was.'

I have always enjoyed being active. It's one of those gifts that one receives without asking for it, and whose value one does not recognize until one is much older. As a child, no one ever needed to tell me to go out and play – I did it of my own volition. I suppose most children are that way – they run, leap, climb, somersault and cartwheel for the pure joy of it, and move as if they had hydraulic springs in their feet. I have been particularly blessed in that the joy I took in activity as a child never quite faded as I grew up.

It helped that the ecosystem in Glasgow, where I was

born, and later in Hertfordshire, where we moved for my dad's job, was entirely supportive of an active lifestyle. My family invariably lived in homes with large gardens. We were walked to school, and had enough unstructured, unsupervised time each afternoon and evening to do as we wished. There were no after-school classes, no sports coaching, no family events to attend and no friends to hang out with. My playmates were my sisters, and I could not have asked for more or better company.

We hardly ever saw Baba during the week – in my memory, he was always working. Aai was the one who raised us, cooking every single one of our meals herself. 'Outside food' was anathema to her; both she and Baba actively discouraged us from buying candy or fizzy drinks like our schoolfellows did. It may have been that there wasn't a lot of money to go around then, especially with four children to care for, but I think it was more Aai's deep distrust of anything that wasn't cooked under her supervision. To this day, she behaves as if restaurants are dens of vice and everything served up in them the equivalent of poison.

These days, despite her continued protestations, my sisters, Ankita and I force her into restaurants for occasional family dinners – all my sisters live in Mumbai, and one of my brothers-in-law runs his own restaurant, so such outings are not uncommon. But as children, we did not mind not eating out – it wasn't a big part of British culture in the '60s for families to eat out, and in any case, Aai's food was far more delicious than anything Britain had to offer.

I was a quiet, serious child, and a bit of a misfit in my almost all-white kindergarten class. Animals, especially injured, abandoned ones that needed care, became my refuge. I was always bringing animals home, but my fondest memory is of my first real pet, a rabbit I named Benjamin. Tragically, he wandered out of his hutch into the snow of an English winter one night and froze to death. My other refuge was reading. That was very much part of British culture, and Aai and Baba approved entirely, being big readers themselves. With my nerd glasses on (I have been short-sighted for most of my life), I dove happily into the seemingly endless sea of children's books – Enid Blyton was a perennial favourite with my sisters and me – available to eager readers in public libraries and at school, and was enriched in ways I could not even articulate. Of all the pursuits available to a quiet, solitary child, reading, apart from being a portal to knowledge, a lesson in empathy and a spur to the imagination, is certainly the most absorbing.

Our weekends were glorious. My best memories are of drives into the English countryside, picnics, chasing butterflies and dragonflies, and wading into ponds and streams with a jam jar to catch fish to bring home. Most of the fish I caught ended up dying within a couple of days, but the joy of making them mine even for a bit was so great that I didn't stop. Even when we returned to live in Bombay, I would wade into gutters to catch fish. I would chase cats, climb walls, run wild in the neighbourhood. Neither Aai nor Baba ever came in the way of the little amusements I fashioned for myself – they were fond of animals as well, and I suppose they could see that my interest in little critters came from a place of curiosity and affection, so they wisely let me be. That ability to let her children be, to support them while letting them explore their individual interests, even if they aren't things she understands or entirely approves of, is something Aai particularly has, in spades. I admire that quality, and as her child, am very grateful for it.

When I was seven, we moved back to Bombay, leaving a wonderful life behind in England. I suppose it wasn't as wonderful for Aai as it was for us children – it could not have been easy for her to manage four children on her own – but she has never been the complaining type and seemed just as happy in England as she was in Bombay. It was different for me, though – I had only been to India once previously, as a child of two, so the 'homecoming' was quite traumatic.

Everything about Bombay was different from what I had known – the number of people and the level of noise around me, the Indian-style toilets, apartment living and, worst of all, a new, unfamiliar school, a boys-only school to boot. To add to my woes, the home we moved to was bang in the middle of Shivaji Park, a middle-class, conservative, Marathi neighbourhood and a Shiv Sena stronghold – i.e., a very different kettle of fish from England, where no one knew enough about us or the culture we came from to expect us to conform in any way; we were simply weird foreigners who were expected to do things differently.

My alma mater, Antonio da Silva High School, was not too far away, in another middle-class Marathi neighbourhood, Dadar. With my close-cropped hair, sticky-out ears, 'Gandhi' glasses and 'posh' foreign accent, I was a ripe target for bullying. Packs of boys I did not know would routinely jump me around corners and try to beat me up or snatch my glasses away. That period did not last, however – unfortunately for my tormentors, I was strong for my age, and knew how to immobilize my adversaries with a wrestling hold or two. More frustratingly for them, I never displayed anger or fear, which would have made the game interesting and given them the high they were looking for. I did not snitch on them to the teachers either, so they had no good reason to gang up against me.

The bullies could not understand why I wasn't reacting in the 'normal' ways. I suppose it was because I realized instinctively, despite being so young, that this would only prolong my engagement with them, when all I wanted was to be left alone. Eventually, out of sheer boredom and incomprehension, they stopped bothering me.

That episode taught me a great lesson for life. If you have clarity on what you want – in my case, at that point, it was solitude – you can focus on that, instead of the stuff that is happening to you and around you. Without such clarity, you will invariably be pulled into your own or someone else's drama and get derailed from where you are headed. As a boy at school, it was instinct that guided my behaviour. As an adult, I do this consciously.

'I started swimming because there was a pool in the neighbourhood and my parents wanted to keep me out of mischief. It was the making of me.'

The school bullies had left me alone, but I was still on the lookout for a sanctuary where I could hide without attracting attention. Naturally, I gravitated to the school library, where I found refuge in a shelf of books, starring Tarzan the Ape Man, by the brilliant Edgar Rice Burroughs. I was captivated by the series from the very first page. In two ticks, I was running, leaping and swinging from vine to vine alongside the magnificent, noble 'Lord of the Apes', learning from him what 'being a man' meant in the jungle that was the world.

People may scoff at this, arguing that Burroughs' first Tarzan story was published in 1912, when ideas of manhood were very different. I would disagree – the most enduring stories are those that appeal to our best selves, inspiring us to respond with courage and compassion in every situation, always believing that we have it in us to overcome any setback, whatever our gender, whatever the times we live in. Tarzan fell squarely in this category. What I had learnt serendipitously during my episode with the bullies – clarity of thought is everything, and it comes from putting emotion aside – was validated by Tarzan in every story, his swift, sure ways of dispensing justice to those who broke the jungle code resonating deeply with me. I don't know about Burroughs' other young readers, but for me, Tarzan, Lord Greystroke, was the hero I wanted to emulate.

While Tarzan fired my imagination and gave me an adrenaline rush, I also craved activity in the real world around me. My desire for solitude ensured that I disliked – and still do – any form of team sport, so I did not try out for the school football, cricket or hockey teams, leaving my evenings free. Recognizing my restlessness, Baba lost no time in enrolling me in the local cadre of the Rashtriya Swayamsevak Sangh (RSS), which had a shakha in Shivaji

Park. Like many Marathi men, he had been part of the RSS himself as a young man, and believed it was a good place for boys to spend time gainfully each evening, being physically active, and learning about disciplined living and moral values through the stories of gods, kings and heroes of the freedom struggle. I was very annoyed when I found out he had signed me up for the organization – I had been trying so hard to avoid activities that involved other boys, and here I was, forced to spend an hour each evening with a bunch of them, just because Baba had decided it was good for me.

In defiance, for the first couple of weeks, I would head out to the shakha at the designated time, but hide out on the sidelines, watching the others. Caught in the act soon after, I resigned myself to my fate with none-too-good grace and began to attend the classes regularly. I can't say I learnt very much about anything at the shakha, but my time there did give me an appreciation of, and love for, Shivaji Park – the big maidan after which the neighbourhood is named – and of all the people who used it for so many different activities. To this day, since I still live in the same house, I do my morning pull-ups on the bar at the outdoor gym at the Park.

Around the same time – I must have been nine then – my parents also enrolled my sisters and me at the Mahatma Gandhi Swimming Pool, an Olympic-sized community pool located around the corner from where we lived. For some reason, my initial, ineffectual flailing on the very crowded, shallow side of the pool caught the attention of the coach, Percy Hakim. He suggested I sign up for coaching classes, dangling the carrot of a dedicated strip of pool for his students during the less-crowded 'Ladies' Time.' I did, and learnt to swim. I would not stop swimming for the next 14 years.

Coach Hakim's somewhat rudimentary methods of training – the order 'Keep Swimming!', barked at us ad nauseam, was really the extent of it – left much to be desired, but it got results. In less than a year after I first learnt to swim, I won a silver medal at the national championships, in the under-11 category. Even though I would not win a medal of any colour again at the national level until I was 15, I kept going.

Two hours at the very least in the pool each day, swimming and swimming and swimming, was a punishing routine for a child, and I marvel that I did it, for so long, without protest, especially since I did not particularly enjoy swimming. Thinking back, I probably would have dropped out at some point if I hadn't won that first medal. For while it was true that I did not enjoy swimming, and had not entered the pool by choice, I certainly, back then, enjoyed winning. Even if I wasn't among the medal winners at the national level between ages 11 and 15, I was at the state level, and that was incentive enough.

Swimming was also, although I didn't think of it that way then, an activity tailor-made for me. Even though I always trained with a large bunch of people, I did not have to interact with them too much – when your face is in the water, there is very little need, or opportunity, for conversation. My swimming routine helped me believe that I was constantly working towards something – the next championship, the next win – and filled my days with structure and purpose. I know that modern educationists believe that too much structure makes robots out of children, and does not allow them to give free rein to their imaginations, but as with other things like fitness regimens, food and medicine, what suits one child may not suit another. I certainly benefited from structure, and I can say with conviction that my structured childhood – and adolescence – did not affect my ability or my eagerness to seek out and explore unconventional paths in later years.

In any case, what would I have done with my time if I wasn't swimming? Unlike others of my age, I did not enjoy playing cricket or sitting on compound walls with other kids, shooting the breeze, watching the world go by. My family did not own a television – Baba gave away our TV set within a year of us moving to Bombay, and we did not have one again until I turned 30, when I bought one for Aai so that she could watch me in a television show. I wasn't given pocket money, so there was no incentive to check out the shops.

There was another thing. My sisters were also swimming competitively, and winning races themselves, which meant they were training each day as well. If they had been playing board games at home, or lolling about reading, I may have resented the daily slog in the pool. But swimming was something we all did as a family – Aai chaperoning us to championships in other cities as and when required, and the rest of us doing it as part of our daily lives, a routine as commonplace as going to school.

Like everything else, a lifetime of good health – physical, mental, spiritual – begins in the home of your childhood. But it is also never too late for anyone to begin the journey to well-being by themselves. Ask yourself what well-being means to you, and why you want it, and then, like the ad line goes, just do it.

ANKITA

My North Lakhimpur Childhood

'I always knew where the food I was eating came from. I believe that cultivating this awareness leads to a deep respect and gratitude, both for the food and its producer. There is no better tonic for good health than gratitude.'

If Salman Rushdie is Midnight's Child by virtue of being born in the year of our independence, I suppose you could call me liberalization's child. I was born in August 1991, right after our then finance minister, Dr Manmohan Singh, took steps to unshackle the Indian economy and set us on a new path. The decade that followed saw urban India explode into free-market consumerism. An entire generation of children were introduced to glitzy malls, international brands, the World Wide Web and the delights of cable TV and American fast food, by indulgent parents with way higher disposable incomes than the generation before.

Not me, though, nor my older sister, Maina, growing up as we did in the small, remote town of North Lakhimpur, some 400 kilometres northeast of Guwahati, just a stone's throw from Assam's border with Arunachal Pradesh. My father, Nagen Chandra Konwar, was a Block Development Officer in charge of Dhemaji district, an hour further northeast by road, by the mighty Brahmaputra. My mother, Niranjana, was a full-time mum, enjoying her hobbies – a bit of stitching, knitting and crochet – when she had some spare time. At home, Papa was a keen gardener, tending lovingly to his vegetable patch and his flowerbeds, an indulgent husband to mum, who he believed needed taking care of, and an enlightened dad who empowered his daughters instead of holding them back. At work, he was an upright, honest officer, and as you can imagine, that got him transferred a lot. That meant we were moved around a lot too, whether we liked it or not.

The one unchanging part of my childhood, the annual ritual that grounded me, was summer vacations spent at my maternal grandparents' home, in a village about 40 kilometres from Lakhimpur. My grandfather (who I called Putha, a shorter, more affectionate version of Puthadeo, the Ahom word for maternal grandfather) owned acres and acres of paddy and mustard fields, and because Assam is one of the few states in India that has three rice-growing seasons, it seemed like it was always harvest time there. After a hard day's work of harvesting, when he had distributed to each worker his share of the harvest, Putha and the rest of the family would sit down with the farmhands to enjoy a hearty dinner. As for my sister and me, we grew up playing with the workers' children and eating the food they ate.

My family and I are proud Ahoms who come from a martial and agrarian lineage, descendants of the Tai people, who arrived at the Brahmaputra valley in the first half of the thirteenth century. Led by the great Chaolung Sukaphaa, who founded the Ahom kingdom in 1228, the Tais brought superior techniques of wet-rice cultivation from China's Yunnan province with them, established their rule over Assam for almost 600 years, and brought the fallow land to the south of the Brahmaputra and the east of the Dikho river under the plough. Over the centuries, they intermarried with the local people and brought local tribes into their fold, creating the state of Assam. In the mid-sixteenth century, the Ahoms came under Hindu influence, and have since followed Hindu social and religious practices.

I myself was raised Hindu – Papa taught my sister and me to chant mantras, Mamma performed her daily pooja, Putha began his day with suryanamaskars and a ritual bath, which involved pouring seven copper buckets of cold water on himself. But the concept of ritual food purity and eating separately from people of other castes was entirely alien to my family. When I first found out about it, in my teens, I don't remember feeling anger at the unfairness of it; instead, my reaction was pure bewilderment – I simply did not get it, because I had never been exposed to such ideas.

The long, hot summer days at Putha's farm were idyllic. With no one monitoring my movements between mealtimes, I ran wild and free. Climbing trees, paddling in the river (I was never taught to swim as a child, but I managed to stay afloat), off-roading on my bicycle, playing cricket all day long, I was forever one of the boys, and anyone who suggested that I behave 'like a girl' was sure to get a dose of my quick temper. Putha was a great one for planting trees, and because I always wanted to do what he was doing, that became one of my favourite activities as well. The farm teemed with snakes and leeches, but I loved being barefoot like my playmates; despite Mamma's dire threats and injunctions, footwear was invariably abandoned early in the day.

The best part about spending so much time on the farm was that I was never in doubt, even as a child, where the food I was eating came from. I cannot overstate the importance of this – when you know the animals you are eating, when you have been involved in the growing and harvesting of grain and vegetable, you eat with a deep sense of gratitude, respect and contentment, understanding at a subconscious level that everything on the earth – including the body that you are now feeding – will one day be fed on. It is impossible to feel, then, like so many of us do today, a distrust of what is on our plates. It is that distrust – *Oh my god, I wonder what chemicals are in this food, I wonder if it has been genetically modified in some way, I wonder if this whole wheat bread really is made of whole wheat* – ends up turning even the most nutritious food into poison in our bodies.

In Putha and Enai's (short for Enaideo, the Ahom word for maternal grandmother) yard were chickens and pigs they raised for the table, and a pond full of plump fish. In their vegetable patch grew the staples of Assamese cuisine – potatoes, sweet potatoes, pumpkins – and several other plants whose leaves routinely went into the cooking pot to enhance the nutritional value or taste of the dish being prepared. Putha used to say, with a bit of a swagger, that the only supplies he bought from the market were jaggery, sugar and salt – even the mustard oil we used in our cooking was home-pressed.

I killed my first chicken when I was ten. No one made a big fuss about it. I was old enough, said Putha, and it was time I learnt how to do it myself. I had watched it done for years, and when it was my turn, I did it without hesitation. It was over very quickly. I felt no sadness or disgust, but a glow of pride that I hadn't put the animal through needless pain from a botched-up job. The bonus was that I got first dibs on the chicken's feet, which Enai fried up for me to enjoy as a crunchy side dish – usually, I would have had to fight the other children for it, since each chicken has only two feet!

My sister and I foraged in Putha's yard for other kinds of food as well. Our favourite evening snack was uisiringa – a species of cricket that is common in Assam. Uisiringa make their homes in the ground, and there are always two holes leading into them – one through which the insects enter, and the other through which they leave. I remember pouring water down one of the holes to force the insects out of the other – as they emerged, I would trap them in a glass and then run to Enai, yelling with excitement, begging her to fry them up for me.

My hometown, Lakhimpur, is also famous for another unusual snack, which also happens to be one of my favourites. That snack is an outcome of Lakhimpur being one of Assam's major silk districts, producing yards and yards of golden, royal Muga silk and 'peaceful' Eri silk, the latter produced without violence, each year. The process of spinning silk thread usually involves first boiling the silkworm cocoons with the worms still inside them, so that one can draw out an unbroken, fine filament of silk from the undamaged cocoon, but the clever Eri worms save themselves by spinning a cocoon with short fibres and leaving a hole open at one end from which the moth can emerge. Muga silkworms, however, are traditional in their cocoon-building approach and not many of them, therefore, get a chance to turn into moths. And what do you think happens to all the boiled silkworms left behind after the silk thread has been unravelled? Why, they are tossed together with some chopped onions and chillies, seasoned, and eaten, of course!

Making a meal of bugs and worms may seem unsavoury to people who aren't used to the idea, but as new science tells us, eating insects (like grasshoppers and crickets) and worms (like mealworms), which are rich in protein and minerals, may be one of the big weapons in humanity's collective arsenal to fight climate change. How? If we can get all the protein we need via insects, we can radically decrease meat production, which will free up farmland, currently being used to raise livestock, for growing foodgrains, which will in turn decrease greenhouse emissions! Plus, if you think about it, foraging for insects and eating them soon after adheres to the mantra of eating fresh, local and seasonal, any which way you look at it, haha.

Staying with new food trends and mantras, here's one I would like to entirely refute. If you are one of those who believe that rice and potatoes are the enemy, perish the thought. I firmly believe that the Assamese staples that I grew up on – poita bhat, a fermented rice gruel, and aloo pitika, a simple dish of mashed boiled potatoes, chillies, salt and a dash of mustard oil, are responsible for making me strong. If you are, understandably, feeling a tiny bit sceptical about my strength or fitness – for it is true that I am only 32 and haven't demonstrated good health over decades like Aai has – how's this for a banger fact? **Chaolung Sukaphaa's Ahom descendants, who also subsisted on poita bhat and aloo pitika, held off the mighty Mughals no less than 17 times!!!** Beat that!

'I do not trust easily. Growing up, I was alone a lot, and learnt to trust my own instinct more than anyone else. That is a lonely road to tread, but it makes you strong and self-reliant.'

My childhood may seem idyllic to many, and it was, mostly. But the bright summer days at Putha's farm also had their dark side, even though I did not realize it at the time. I'm not sure if that was a good thing or a bad thing, and I will lay it open for you to decide for yourselves. But first, a little more about my childhood away from the farm.

As I mentioned, Papa used to get transferred a lot, and we moved along with him. This was fine when my sister and I were young, but when his marching orders came along in the summer before Maina went into Grade 9, to a town that had no schools of the standard we had been used to, my parents decided that boarding school was the answer. They picked a school in North Lakhimpur, and both of us were packed off. I was 10 or 11 then, and glad to have my sister with me.

Unfortunately, Maina was not happy at boarding school; she quit the moment she completed her tenth grade. I didn't particularly love the school myself, but I had gotten used to the routine there and didn't want to put myself through another move, so I voted to continue. But perhaps the bigger reason I chose to stay was that I did not want to cause my parents additional stress. This is how I was as a child. I tended not to complain, to make do, to not call attention to myself if I could help it. I was exactly the kind of kid teachers loved – I got good grades and never got into trouble.

However, my reluctance to be a burden ensured that I did not take my problems at school to anyone, least of all my parents. Having to deal with stuff on your own can feel like a lot, and can completely break people – my generation seems particularly susceptible. The prevailing wisdom, dinned into us at every opportunity, is that there is no shame in asking for help when you need it. Of course this is true, but for me, it has always been a case of trying to sort things out in my own head rather than depend overly on advice from friends, family or a therapist. However, learning to trust yourself and your instinct isn't easy, especially when what you feel is at odds with what the rest of the world says you should be feeling. Rest assured that you will have to walk some dark paths to get to that place of light.

I was 14 or 15 when it dawned on me that what I had experienced on Putha's farm when I was about 4 or 5, with his brother's son – my uncle, once removed – was molestation. For a time, I wondered why it had happened to me, why I had been particularly singled out for that kind of violation. I then asked myself what I could do about that, ten years later. I supposed I could mope about it, blame the adults who had failed to protect me, feel bitter and defeated, and decide to hate the world. I sat with that for a bit. But try as I might, I could not see how any of those reactions would help make my life better. I could tell someone in the family what had happened. But what would that achieve? It would only make them feel guilty, helpless and sad.

It was then that I began to take my long, solitary walks and my longer bicycle rides. Sometimes, when the Subansiri river wasn't full, I would cycle all the way to the border of Assam with Arunachal Pradesh, some 40 kilometres away from school – thank you for the genes, Ahom ancestors! – riding the heck out of my basic bicycle on those hilly, unpaved roads. Luckily for me, the supervisor at school was happy to go easy on the older students, so long as we returned to school before curfew. The physical exertion emptied my mind of emotion and allowed me to think clearly. **I realized, subconsciously at first, how inextricably the body and mind were connected, how acutely one influenced the other.** Today, it has become a habit that is almost unconscious; whenever I feel overwhelmed by something and need clarity, I go for a run.

A few years later, a solution that I felt comfortable with showed up – I decided to talk about my childhood experience of abuse. I knew by then that many, many children had experienced such abuse, almost always perpetrated by a close family member. Well then, by talking about it, I would help parents and grandparents better protect the children in their care, and help children protect themselves. Remarkably, I never felt any shame about what had happened to me, which I may have if I had shared my thoughts with anyone else – so often, it is other people's reactions to situations that fashion our own.

Life is neither good nor bad, just a series of experiences that we live through. Sometimes we embrace the bright side, sometimes the dark, but what is important is that we tell ourselves, each time – This is an *experience*, it is *not* my life. I believe I came to this realization early simply because I was alone so much, and the solitude taught me how to commune with myself. I know it may not work for everyone, and I would never judge anyone for finding other ways to cope, but **I believe it was this ability to draw strength from myself, and the early lessons I learnt, serendipitously, on how I could use physical activity to get to mental fitness, that would pull me through the massive setbacks that awaited me further down the road.**

THE SOMAN SUTRA: HOW TO BUILD AN ACTIVE FAMILY

Usha: Don't focus too much on your child's academic performance, especially when they're young. Focus equally on physical activity – it not only fills out a child's personality but also sends out a crucial message: coming first in class isn't everything. Children are naturally active; all you need to do as a parent is to validate this. Learn and/or play a sport together, formally – it will help you both.

Milind: Only one rule: use technology as an intervention, only when critically needed. As a family, take the lift only if you cannot climb the stairs for some reason. Walk if your destination is within a 1.5 kilometre radius, instead of taking the car. Use a calculator only when the math is complicated. Try to recall who directed that film instead of Googling it instantly. Get the app that tracks your daily screentime – and set a time limit for yourself. Reduce tech, and you are automatically more active, physically and mentally.

Ankita: Make a game out of your workout routine so that the kids join in without your urging. Send the children out for groceries. Race them up the stairs. Kick a football around in the evenings. Try and make at least 50% of family time active time instead of always plumping for movie night with double-butter popcorn.

THE SOMAN SUTRA: HOW TO RAISE AN EMPOWERED CHILD

Usha: Literally and metaphorically, once your child starts walking, let go of their hand. It isn't easy to stand by and watch your children struggle or make choices that you believe are unwise, but bite your tongue. Stay alert and watchful, but do it subtly. When they do ask for help, *if* they ask for it, support them in every way you can. Eventually, your child will come to trust their own instincts, which is the best outcome for them.

Milind: Haha, how would I know? But if I ever had to, I would raise my children like my mother raised me. I would adopt, like her, a 'Show, don't tell' style of parenting – I saw Aai being extremely hard-working, uncomplaining, positive and supportive of her family, and those became my values as well. Be non-judgemental companions to your kids, not their supervisors – that will make them fearless about trying new things and indifferent to failure.

Ankita: Guide your children, but don't force-fit them into your expectations – they are their own people, with their own talents, drawbacks and destinies. My father, who was my biggest emotional support, used to say, 'I will accept whatever you decide, but if your decision turns out to be a mistake, you will have to clean up your own mess.' I was grateful for the freedom that he gave me, but the latter part of the statement made me consider each of my decisions very carefully.

SECTION 2

TAKING CHARGE

Falling, Learning, Adapting, Evolving

What is adulting, really? How much does it have to do with age, and how much with developing the ability to accept setbacks with grace and equanimity, before finding the courage to pick yourself up, dust yourself off and go back to start in good heart, determined to try again? Is it about finally reaching the tipping point at which you stop blaming your parents, your partner, your children and your circumstances for the challenges that confront you at every turn, and choose consciously, emphatically, relentlessly, to stop casting yourself as a victim? Perhaps it happens when you finally begin to see yourself as whole, powerful and independent, and forge ahead, free of anxiety, full of love for yourself and the world, to fashion and take charge of your own physical, mental and spiritual destiny.

USHA

Fashioning a Fulfilling Life Out of a Challenging One

'Finding my feet in Glasgow among people who automatically believed they were superior to me wasn't easy. My breakthrough was realizing that their behaviour was driven by ignorance – theirs, not mine.'

I was married, at 21, to Prabhakar Soman, a 26-year-old pharmacologist. His family were Kokanastha Brahmins from the Alibag area, and strictly vegetarian, at least at home. Unlike my own family, they were also more chapati-eaters than rice-eaters. Since I was going to live with them, I was forced to turn vegetarian myself, and also eat far less rice than I was used to. That adjustment was very difficult for me in the beginning, but there was no way out, so I went with it.

Just like me, my husband had a parent and a step-parent who were doctors – seriously, what are the odds? My father-in-law had struggled to put himself through medical school in India and the UK, becoming a husband and father along the way. When his wife died young, leaving him with three children to take care of, he got married again, to a young doctor. When I first met her, she was a professor at the JJ Medical College. It was she my husband considered his mother.

In 1961, just a year after my marriage, I gave birth to my first child, a daughter, who we named Netra. A few months later, my husband was offered a seat in the pharmacology master's programme at the University of Strathclyde in Glasgow, and decided to take it. I had an infant in my care and my own master's degree in biochemistry to complete, so I stayed back in Bombay.

Finances were tight, what with my husband himself being on a student allowance, which the Reserve Bank of India (RBI) did not allow him to repatriate to India. What's more, once he had gotten to university, he had decided to pursue a combined master's and PhD programme, which meant that the state of our finances wasn't about to change significantly any time soon. I was educated, I told myself; surely I could find some work in Glasgow to support us! In 1962, I left for the UK, leaving Netra in my mother's care. I would not be back, even for a visit, for the next four years – people did not traipse back and forth across continents on a whim then, as they do now. It was hard on me and hard on the child – Netra took a while to get over the fact that she had been 'left behind'. Fortunately for me, she did not cling to her sense of hurt. Today, we are the best of friends.

Those four years were quite the challenge, but Britain was also the making of me. In my marital home, I had gotten used to having a cook around – my mother-in-law, being a working woman, had always had one. And dear, dear Bombay, which had always been home, was familiar, comfortable, a place I knew my way around. All of a sudden, I had been pitched into an alien land where I knew not a soul. For the first time in my life, I was entirely on my own, negotiating spaces populated by people who believed they were superior to me. I had to fend for myself and take charge of my life, because there was no one there who would do it for me. There were some silver linings – my husband had begun to eat meat in Britain, so I could go back to eating the food I was raised on. Buoyed by this and other small triumphs, I learnt to drive, got a job in a research institute and began to hone my English.

I knew English, of course, but wasn't as fluent in it conversationally as I am now, and I was very conscious of this prominent marker of my 'otherness'. Many of the people

I met and interacted with in the UK were kind, but there were also those to whom my level of education mattered not a whit; they simply assumed, because of my halting English, that I was ignorant. What they did not realize was that I would eventually draw my strength from their own deeper ignorance, which had been revealed to me by their snobbery and standoffishness. I understood how backward *they* were in their inability to 'see' others for who they really were, people just like themselves, made up of equal parts of hope and love and fear. The moment I had this epiphany, my anxiety and awkwardness disappeared.

This unexpected, serendipitous insight into an ignorant person's mind that I received then has stood me in good stead through my life; it has given me the mental and emotional fortitude – both of which count hugely towards 'good health' in my books – to face new and challenging situations with composure and equanimity. I have learnt that **if you are able to confront such situations without being burdened by your own sense of perceived injury or betrayal, life's curveballs, whenever they come, cannot faze you.**

'I travelled alone from Bombay to London in 1967 with four children under six. This is what I learnt from the experience: don't say "I can't do it" without trying something, because you do not know your own abilities.'

In my first four-year stint in the UK, I would not only hold down a few jobs but also give birth to two more children – Medha in 1964 and Milind in 1965. Through it all, however, I never stopped working, thanks to my wonderful babysitter – a white woman married to a Pakistani man – who took very good care of my babies. In 1966, my husband completed his PhD and got a job at the pharmaceutical giant Smith, Kline and French (SKF) in Hertfordshire. Reassured that things would be easier and more stable now, I quit my job as a biochemist in a nearby hospital and took a ship back home from Marseilles, pregnant again and with two toddlers in tow, telling my husband I'd be back once he had settled down in his job and set up some kind of home for us. It was a cargo-cum-passenger ship we travelled by, and the journey took close to two weeks, with stops at ports on the way.

Six months later, once our home was ready, I made my way back to the UK, this time as the sole chaperone of *four* children (for I was also taking Netra back with me this time) below the age of six; the youngest, Anupama, was still a babe in arms. Looking back, I marvel at my own strength and courage; I wonder how I did it all, and all alone. **But sometimes the best, even the only, way to truly understand what you are capable of is to be challenged.**

Despite my husband always being very busy at work, and having very little time for the family, our life in England proceeded enjoyably enough. Sure, with four children on my hands, it was difficult for me to do much more than make sure they were dressed and fed and sent to school on time. But the very fact that there were four of them worked to my advantage, and theirs, for they never needed any playmates other than each other. Plus, our house had a large garden, where the children, and any pets we had at the time (including Benjamin, Milind's rabbit), could run free. The evenings followed a simple, set routine – the kids would eat their after-school snack, watch a children's programme on TV for about half an hour, and then go out to play in the garden. Dinner was around 7.30 p.m. on schoolnights, after which they would go to their room and amuse themselves with board games or reading until it was time for bed.

With the children's school and my husband's work, outings were not that frequent. But when he could get away, my husband would drive all of us to some nice outdoor location – the seashore, a petting zoo, a hillside covered in flowers. We would carry a picnic basket full of food and make a day of it. Once again, what worked to our advantage was that the children had each other's company.

It was a simple, lovely life, but because my husband eventually wanted to go back to India, we knew that life was only temporary. Perhaps it was that knowledge that made us cherish those years more.

In 1972, my husband landed a job with the Bhabha Atomic Research Centre in Bombay. We returned to our home with joy, and a wee bit of trepidation – Netra was of course a Bombay girl, but Anupama had left when she was three months old and had no knowledge of India. As for Medha and Milind, they hadn't been 'home' for over five years. I knew it would be unsettling for them, but there was nothing to be done about it. I would just have to lead the way and hope that they would cope.

I must mention something here that I personally find rather remarkable. When I say we returned 'home', I don't mean it only in the sense of city or country or community – I mean a specific physical space. In 1944, my father-in-law rented an apartment in Shivaji Park and moved his family into it. That was the home I went into as a young bride in 1960. In 1972, we returned with our own young family to the same two-bedroom, first-floor apartment. At the time, the second bedroom was small, almost a passage, but the kitchen, tucked away at one end of the house, was large.

Conveniently so, for there were often eight people to be fed – our family of six, and my in-laws, who stayed for months when they visited. And there was the one bathroom that we all shared. By today's standards, it would be considered too small for eight people, but we didn't feel constrained. My daughters' friends often stayed over, too, and it was never a problem – mattresses were rolled out on the floor and everyone was accommodated.

Now that there are only three of us living here, the house has been remodelled. The kitchen is smaller, the bedrooms are bigger, there is a second bathroom – it is all very convenient. The remarkable part is that 80 years after it was first rented by a Soman, it is still a Soman who is paying the rent!

I don't know what that says about us as a family, but this state of affairs suits me very well. We are lucky of course, in a city as space-constrained as Mumbai, to have had this well-located roof over our heads for generations, but honestly, I would not move even if 'better' options came along. I don't quite understand the fascination for travel or movement for no strong reason that people today have in such extravagant measure.

Maybe it's the mindset I grew up with. When we were young, and even when the children were young, most travel was for pilgrimage – people went on yatras, and the whole thing, from start to finish, was seen as a necessary spiritual journey that enhanced the quality of one's inner life. No doubt I crossed the seas to support my husband's professional ambitions, but I have been more than content to stay put after that. It is only in the past couple of decades, post my retirement, that I have learnt – more correctly, 'been taught to' – appreciate the pleasures of 'travel for leisure'. I travel quite a bit with Milind and Ankita now, and enjoy it, because it usually involves some kind of physical activity in the lap of nature.

I do know what the fact that we have lived here for so many years says about the *house*, though – it has good bones. My brother Vinayak, the civil engineer, says that this is true of many older buildings in Bombay; they are solidly constructed. It also says something about a way of life that is now well and truly behind us. In my time, most people lived in the same house, and worked in the same job, throughout their lives. Today's generation may well scoff at that, and ask – how can one be content living or working in the same place year after year when the world has so much to offer and life is so short? How can you be happy doing what you are doing now and being who you are today for the rest of your life, when you can do and be so many other things as well? What kind of life is it that does not have the excitement of the new at every turn?

Here's my answer: a rooted, steady life, a life in which one finds joy in what one already has, learns to appreciate it more each day by examining it minutely, and nourishes it while being nourished by it. And that is as true of houses and it is of our own bodies – instead of chasing after what the world tells you is an ideal body, or a better life, I believe it is important to heartily embrace the one you have been gifted. Take the effort to build a relationship with what you have, so that you intimately understand its workings, and treat it as it deserves to be treated – exactly like you would your most favourite, most valuable, most irreplaceable possession. **Put time, patience, discipline and love into building the edifice of your body, and your life, around 'good bones', and you will never have cause for regret.**

'Good health can be cultivated. Genetics play a part, but if you know what conditions you have a predisposition for, you can take care of it.'

My husband was very much into bodybuilding. He was a very strong man and had great respect and admiration for sportspeople. In the early days of our marriage, I noticed that he slept very deeply, abnormally so, especially after a heavy meal. That tipped me off that something was wrong. I had him go for a couple of tests, which revealed that he was a juvenile diabetic. It was a huge shock to him to discover that he was not in the best health despite his youth and his wholesome lifestyle. The condition was probably something he carried in his genes, though – his own mother had died young, of causes no one had bothered to investigate too deeply, so there was no way of knowing if she had passed it on to him.

He was immediately put on insulin, which he stubbornly resisted – despite being from a family of doctors, he had always hated consulting doctors. Instead, since he was a trained pharmacologist, he decided he would take care of himself. I have to say he did that very well. He took every precaution to stay healthy and monitored his own doses of medication till the last. Later in life, he also had heart trouble; I am not sure if this was because of his temper or his genetic makeup. But watching him take such good care of himself made me see that **good health is also the result of a strong desire for it, and the will to make it so, whatever the discipline and sacrifices it demands.**

'My husband and I never had much use for religion or rituals, and the children picked up on that. What they also picked up on was our love for the outdoors, and the joy that comes from being active. I think those are great gifts to give your children.'

As a girl, I used to enjoy going to temples. My father was a great believer in God and rituals, so there was always a lot of it going on around me. My siblings still follow some of those traditions in their own homes and families. As for me, I have always been the unusual one, questioning everything. I have been the one that read books, observed people, listened to their conversations and then made up my own mind – whatever the subject.

On the subject of religion, I wondered as a teenager why people who insisted that God was everywhere were so hell-bent on rushing around from temple to temple. I wondered why one had to pay a priest to perform a standard ritual; as I understood it, there was no standard practice when it came to God. A devotee could offer anything that they wanted, out of love or gratitude, in their own way. They certainly did not have to resort to a middleman to facilitate it for them. But that was what temples were all about. Slowly, I stopped going; sometimes, when I feel like it, I go to a small shrine and make an offering.

There was another thing. My husband wasn't a religious person as a young man (in later life, he took a 180 degree turn and became deeply interested in adhyatma or spirituality). The elders in the family I married into were not into mainstream religious practices either, which made it easier for me to remain who I was. My mother-in-law was an adherent of the Prarthana Samaj, a social and religious reform movement founded in 1867 in Maharashtra. Members of the Samaj were big believers in God, but in the great traditions of Namdev and Tukaram, they worshipped a formless God – no idols for them! My father-in-law eventually joined her.

When I moved to Glasgow, I got so busy with children, work and housework, all of which was new to me, that there was really no time to do a puja each day in the way I would have liked. My priorities changed; I stopped feeling the vibe. In the end, I stopped doing the rituals entirely.

I do believe in a power greater than us that we can harness to make our lives better, calmer, more rewarding and less stressful, but I don't believe one has to visit temples or perform rituals to access it – one simply has to look within.

Naturally, since they were raised by parents who weren't much into God, ritual or religion, my children are not into any of it themselves. But since those same parents enjoyed being outdoors and were physically active, all four continue to be active and fit to this day and retain a deep love for nature.

Did we as parents push our children towards formalized physical activity, like football or cricket or swimming? Not when they were very young – they took no such classes at all in England. By the time we moved back to the Bombay flat, however, they were all a little older. I had help, both from my in-laws and from domestic helpers. There was no garden the kids could play in, and so, for the first time, I began to think of other ways to occupy them.

Luckily for us, the Olympic-sized Mahatma Gandhi Swimming Pool in Shivaji Park was just around the corner from our home. I suppose I could have enrolled the children in music or dance lessons, but swimming seemed the most appealing simply because it was so convenient. Plus, all of them took to it quite happily. Without wasting any time, I signed the children up for after-school lessons. As it turned out, all four of them went on to swim competitively at some point in their lives – Netra and Anupama represented Maharashtra for a while, and Milind, who became the Indian Men's 100 metre breaststroke champion at the age of 18, defended his title successfully for the next four years.

Meanwhile, animals, who had been part of our life in England, continued to find their way home to us. My husband was as fond of animals as the rest of us, so he had no objection to the menagerie at all. Someone was once looking to find a family for a star tortoise they had brought home from the Konkan coast, since they could not figure out how to take care of it themselves, and our neighbours gladly volunteered our home as the perfect place. That was how Ruby came into our lives, almost as soon as we had moved back. She lived for 18 long years – she may have lived much longer in the wild – and was a dear companion to all my children in their younger days. She was also the neighbourhood's star attraction – children were always coming up to see her and feed her spinach, coriander leaves and slices of apple. Star tortoises are now classified as a vulnerable species, and you could be penalized if you kept them as pets, but there was no such thing in the '70s and '80s.

Each set of parents – and indeed, each individual parent – passes on a set of unsolicited gifts to their offspring, some beneficial, some patently not so. If I had to pick a gift I am truly happy to have passed on, it is the love for the outdoors and the joy that comes from being active, if only because I can see how well, and in how many different ways, it has sustained each of my children.

THE THING ABOUT AAI

Aai does a *lot* for someone over 80. She is *always* pushing her boundaries. If you say 'Don't do it, it may be too much for you', you can be sure she will.

But Aai doesn't do things to prove something to the world. She does them because she truly believes that is the way to stay healthy. If I am feeling under the weather myself, I prefer to recover by resting. A lot! A recent bout of flu really laid me low – I was exhausted. I could feel that my body needed rest. And what was Aai's genuine, well-meaning advice? 'I'm telling you, Ankita, go for a walk. Movement – that's what will make you better.' Are you serious, Aai??

No matter how much I rib her, and how exasperated I sometimes behave at her refusal to take it easy, I have nothing but admiration for Aai's determination and resilience. Her self-belief is so strong that it helps her get past any physical difficulty she may feel. It is true that she continues to be physically fit because of her lifestyle, but it is her tremendous mental strength that I really envy.

– Ankita

Aai is a pragmatist. One of the credos she lives by is 'it is what it is'. That's probably why she has always gotten on so well with all my girlfriends, and why she accepted my wife so warmly. But her brand of what some people may call fatalism is not a passive, resigned acceptance of her situation; it is a potent combination of calm acceptance, a refusal to take things personally (which allows her to examine whatever it is with dispassion and deal with it without anger or resentment), and the will to get through the hardship in a way that causes the least distress to everyone involved. She doesn't see herself as a martyr for living this way, she does it for a selfish reason – her own peace of mind.

I have grown up around this kind of energy all my life, and some of that attitude has certainly come down to me. But if you asked me what I would really want that is Aai's, her outlook on life would not be at the top of my wish list. What I really want her to leave to me in her will – and I've said this to her many times – are her knees. They've clocked thousands of kilometres of walking and moving in their lives and are still going strong!

– Milind

MILIND

From Straying Off the Path to Finding My Way Back

'For a most productive life, to enjoy what you do as much as possible for as long as possible, there is only one shortcut, and that is consistency. Do something towards a fit, healthy life every single day, and it will change you, shape you, become you.'

At the age of 15, after not winning any medals for four years, I started making my way back to the podium at the national level. As I began to show greater promise, I was plucked out of my laid-back Shivaji Park pool and brought in to train at the posh Otter's Club in Bandra, where the best of the Maharashtra swimmers trained, under a coach far more professional than Percy Hakim. If I had believed Coach

Hakim's coaching was brutal, things were about to get far, far worse, and at very many levels.

For one, everything about the boys I had trained with in Shivaji Park – their accents, clothes, concerns, lifestyles, the amount of money they had, how they spent their time – was different from the Bandra set I was now hobnobbing with. I had only crossed the Mahim Creek, but I might as well have landed on an alien planet. In Antonio da Silva, when I had first arrived, I had been the posh 'English' boy from London; now, I was its polar opposite – the Marathi boy from the boonies.

At home, gentle murmurs of disapproval were beginning to surface about how much time I was devoting to swimming. I had just finished Grade 10, and my paternal grandfather thought it was time I quit the intensive training and focused on my academics. His concerns were understandable – I came from a family of professionals. From my grandparents downwards, even the women had degrees in medicine or science. Plus, I was that rare thing in my family – a boy. There was no such thing then as a 'career in sport' as there is now – it was all far too risky. More importantly, with the New Delhi Asian Games less than two years away, training was bound to get more stringent, especially if I got picked for the national camp. The Games were scheduled for

November 1982, mere months before I sat my Grade 12 boards.

I understood the concern, but was very, very reluctant to give it all up just when all those years of hard work were beginning to bear fruit. Luckily, my parents themselves did not insist that I give up just yet. Baba was very proud of my sporting achievements, and Aai was happy to support me in whatever I wanted to do. But Baba and I did not have the best relationship otherwise – he was opinionated, often angry (mostly at his own bad health, which he took out on people around him), and had allowed himself to get bitter and resentful. As a hot-headed teenager, my responses to him weren't always the most calibrated, leading to a tense atmosphere at home.

Against this background, it was more swimming, not less, that I saw as my refuge. Swimming allowed me to stay out of the house – and the arguments – for several hours a day, especially with the added commute to and from Bandra. At the end of each day, I tumbled into bed, and instantly fell into deep, dreamless sleep, completely exhausted – there was not even enough energy left to sustain a sulk, let alone full-blown anger.

This is one of the great benefits of physical exercise. Any low-grade emotional or mental stress that we are carrying – and we are all carrying some measure of both on most days – can be whittled down and purged through the body by the simple expedient of putting it through some curated stress. **Exert your body, in other words, to calm your mind.**

I did not make the cut for the 1982 Asian Games, but I was among the hopefuls picked for the national camp. For the first time, we had a foreign coach looking into our training. Through the techniques he taught us, I learnt how to streamline my stroke and be faster in the water. A year after the Asian Games, at the age of 18, I was crowned National Open Men's Champion in the 100 metre breaststroke. At long last, I was, in my favourite category, the fastest Indian in the water. I would defend my title successfully for the next four years, breaking personal and national records consistently, and easily qualifying for the 1986 Asian Games.

By this time, everyone at home had made peace with my decision to keep swimming, especially after I met them halfway by enrolling in a diploma course in electrical engineering. I was free to focus fully on the Asian Games, and I did, swimming 12 kilometres every single day for two years.

Such consistent, specific exercise over years and years, emphasizing the use of certain muscles over others, and supported by the kind of lung power required by swimmers, sculpts a body in a very specific way. Long-distance runners have a silhouette very different from sprinters, the body of a champion wrestler looks nothing like that of a tae kwon do master. By the time I arrived at the national training camp for the 1986 Asian Games, over ten years after I had first begun to swim, I was a full 6 feet of perfect 'swimmer's body' – shaped like a V from my broad shoulders to my narrow hips. My body at 20 did not look anything like today's aesthetic ideal – a 'gym body', with bulging biceps and six-pack abs (such a body, by the way, is no indicator of its occupant's fitness) – but by God, it was in the best possible shape for doing what it had been trained to do.

I must clarify here that Indian swimmers then had zero chance of winning anything at the Asian Games. We are still to break that barrier – even at the 2023 Asian Games in Hangzhou, no Indian swimmer managed to make it to the podium. But the Australian coach at the national camp leading up to the 1986 Asiad took one look at my physique and said, simply, 'We can do something with this.' I was elated. By some trick of nature or nurture, my body had shaped itself into something that had the potential to be even better than it was at what it had trained for.

When people ask me for tips on staying fit, I tell them that it isn't how many reps of a particular routine you do, what time you wake up, how much time you spend in the gym, what you eat or how much water you drink that help you stay fit and healthy; the only shortcut to fitness is consistency. It is about doing something active, every single day, over and over, until it becomes a habit you cannot break.

—

'All the data and research in the world cannot tell you what food or exercise is right for you – it can only point you in a particular direction. There is no substitute for self-awareness – understanding what works for your body.'

My 20-year-old body had certainly been shaped by movement, but was it also shaped by the food I had eaten over the years? Was it that, by a fluke of geography, cuisine, culture or personal choice, I had consistently consumed a diet more geared to building the perfect swimmer's physique? It would have to have been a fluke, considering that no one in those days talked about special diets, even for champion sportspersons.

Because here's the truth: what I ate, especially in the years of hard swimming, can be summed up in three words – Anything and Everything. I was constantly hungry, and even in a roomful of teenage boys and young men with enormous appetites, mine was the talk of the town. Entire loaves of bread, whole 100 gram packs of Amul butter, mountains of rice, stacks of rotis, chicken, mutton, dal, glasses and glasses of sugar-laden 'juice' made up from instant drink mix – anything that was on the table went down into my black hole of a stomach.

As for sweets – I love sweets – chocolate was, and continues to be, a firm favourite. At home, I used to have an entire shelf of milk chocolate and white chocolate, a remembered taste from my English childhood, that no one else was allowed to touch. A 'sportsman's diet'? Hardly.

In the last 40 years, we have gained tremendous knowledge about the human body and its physiology, and a deeper understanding of how different elements of what we eat affect us. There are wearable devices that monitor our body processes in real time and all kinds of tests to figure out what is going on in our bodies. But the Age of Information is also the Age of Disinformation – all kinds of conflicting theories abound, and one is never sure what to trust or how to analyse all the data that we have access to. The bigger problem is that these theories are based on statistical data, and the human body, much as we would like to believe the opposite, is too unique to fit into this kind of pigeonholing.

What I have learnt in my life as an athlete is that the only data you can really trust with respect to your body is your subjective experience. Keeping up to date with the research is important, because it may help you analyse your own body experience better. But taking the findings as gospel truth, and applying them to yourself blindly, is unwise. What is worse is believing that what worked for someone you admire and want to emulate will also work for you in exactly the same way.

I have no idea how I not only survived but thrived on what I ate as a young swimmer – I can only hazard that it was the intense physical activity I was doing alongside that helped my body digest my food and absorb the nutrition contained in it very efficiently. Plus, it was mostly simple, plain food that I was eating – freshly cooked, nothing too spicy or oily or fatty – even at the training camps.

But just because I was not damaged by gorging on, among other things, white bread and chocolate, does not make them good things for you to eat, especially given how differently food is grown and processed today. It does not even make them good for *me* to eat, at my current age and activity levels, unless my experiments on myself, at 58, tell me so.

—

'When you are thrust into a challenging situation, explore it, engage with it, analyse your response to it. Then, once you have resolved it, let it go.'

The final selections for the 1986 Asiad were nigh. Determined to make the best use of the Australian coach's expertise, I keenly followed his every instruction. This brought me into conflict with the Indian team coach, who, suddenly insecure, was issuing very different instructions. One day, sick of being made a pawn in an ego battle, I let my famous temper rip. 'Please don't interfere in my training,' I said to the Indian coach, momentarily forgetting how much power he had over my future. 'I prefer to follow the instructions of the other coach.'

Retribution was swift. When the final list of swimmers selected to represent India at the Asian Games went up on the board, my name wasn't on it. The dream was over.

It was grossly unjust – by leaving out the reigning national champion from the squad, the officials had made a travesty of the selection process itself. I was furious, disbelieving and devastated by turns. All my years of hard, hard effort in the pool had come to nought – the one chance I had had to represent India at the Asiad was gone, slipping from my hands in the most perverse way possible.

Four years later, I would be too old – as everyone knows, swimming is a young man's game. Worse, I was partly to blame for my situation.

There are many ways you can go after such a disaster. I could have quit swimming in protest. I could have turned bitter and resentful. I could have sworn to myself that I would 'show the Indian coach' by making it to the squad at the next Asiad, and trained with renewed vigour. All of them would have been impulsive, emotional decisions. I chose none of them. Instead, I went back to the one place which allowed my mind to float free, thoughtless, at peace, even as my body performed a punishing, rhythmic, repetitive activity through muscle memory. I went back to the pool with no goals or ambitions, my only purpose being the relentless physical exertion that had been the raison d'être of my life for so many years.

What do you do when you are unexpectedly thrust into a challenging situation? Simply sitting with it, or surrendering to it, is not an option. You have to explore it, engage with it. How do you do that? By observing closely your reactions to the situation and by questioning those reactions to find out what emotion, what fear, is at the root of your particular response.

That was what I was doing in the pool, trying to find the deeper source of my anger and frustration at not making it to the Games. While I plumbed the depths, both literally and figuratively, I won another national championship. That win brought me some closure, but no great joy.

The penny dropped. I realized then that I had allowed swimming, which had been the biggest part of my life for over a dozen years, to become my identity. I had grown too attached to it, even though it was something I had got into without actively choosing to. It had brought me success, given me purpose, taught me discipline and served as sanctuary during my tumultuous teenage years, and I was grateful for all of it. But it did not own me, and I did not need it any more. There were universes beyond swimming waiting to be explored, and I was ready for them.

In 1988, two years after the Asiad debacle, I climbed out of the pool with no regret or bitterness. Once again, simply by acknowledging a stress-making situation while resisting the temptation to respond emotionally to it, I had been able to jettison it from my system and keep moving – swiftly, lightly, without baggage. I hardly swam again for the next 15 years.

'If you want to live life on your own terms, you have to learn to become comfortable with uncertainty. It's the only way.'

I was 23 and had no idea what I was going to do for the rest of my life. I had a diploma in engineering, but did not see myself doing that kind of work. The path that offered itself to me, the opportunity that dropped out of nowhere right into my lap, was one I could not have imagined for myself in my wildest dreams.

It happened this way. One day in 1989, a very good-looking friend of mine, who was also a champion swimmer, asked me if I would do him a favour. He was supposed to audition for a print ad for Graviera Suitings later that day, but would not be able to make it. Would I audition in his place? I had nothing planned for that afternoon, so I agreed. I didn't get the job – the lady running the auditions thought I looked too young to carry off a suit. I shrugged, and did not give it a second thought. Three weeks later, however, she called back, saying she was looking for a model for a shirting campaign for Thackersay Fabrics, and thought I fit that bill perfectly. When I heard how much they were going to pay – fifty thousand rupees!!! – I jumped on board immediately.

This was 1989, years before the internet became accessible to common Indians. Social media, in the form of Facebook, would not arrive until September 2006. The ways of getting to 'famous' in that age were very different from what they are today. Four years as national swimming champion had brought me very little recognition or adulation from the general public. But one ad, featured on a giant billboard outside the old Cadbury House on Bombay's Pedder Road, changed all that.

The real flex happened a few weeks later, when I met a new species of Indian – the Fashion Designer – for the first time. Gudda (Rohit Bal) was only a few years older than I, but he was as different from me as chalk from cheese. He spoke passionately about clothes, using unfamiliar words like silhouette and cut and drape and style. He was launching a new menswear 'collection', whatever that meant, and was looking for fresh faces to model it. Once I was 'approved', he confessed he could not afford to pay me, because he was trying something that hadn't been done before – a fashion show – and had no idea how it would go down.

I was intrigued by this man, his dreams, and his intensity; I wanted to stick around and see what lay on the other side. As I was to discover on the wildest ride of my life, what lay on the other side was money, pan-Indian fame and the kind of wild female adulation that a middle-class boy from Shivaji Park could never have envisioned for himself. Over the course of the next five years, in the same period that Aamir

Khan, Shah Rukh Khan and Salman Khan became national icons, I went from being Milind Soman, unknown champion swimmer, to Milind Soman, celebrity, media darling and India's first-ever male supermodel.

I took to the celeb life like a fish to water. It was new, exciting and glamorous – beautiful clothes, beautiful people, luxurious settings and over-the-top parties where alcohol flowed like water at someone else's expense. I was no longer a sportsman, and I was suddenly feeling the weight of all the years when I had missed out on the normal rites of passage into adulthood because I had been too busy swimming. Add my natural curiosity into the mix and you have a potent cocktail. (The saving grace was that fast bikes and cars, which were the other passions of the swish set I was surrounded by, had never held any charm for me – I still do not drive if I can help it.)

By this time, I had also got into business with my then girlfriend, who was older, more sophisticated, and part of a different social set from mine. In my first crack at entrepreneurship, I became her partner in an event management company that she was the brains of. The one common factor across all the events we managed was easy access to free alcohol. For months, I came home completely smashed several times a week, having consumed, quite often, an entire bottle of hard liquor in an evening. Never one to judge her children's choices, Aai nevertheless indicated her strong disapproval by speaking as little as possible to me, trusting that I would get the hint.

Then there were the drugs. I didn't do the dirty stuff, but I did indulge in my favourites, marijuana and coke. I loved how hyper coke made me, and the calm and (what I thought of as) 'clarity' that a hit of weed brought on. Until, in 1994, I ended up missing a fashion show because I could not move; an afternoon of smoking joints and chewing on hash had left me paralysed where I lay in my room. I was a big draw by then, and the organizers of the show were not pleased in the least. I was awash in guilt and self-loathing. How had I let it come to this?

All the cautionary tales I had ever heard growing up, at home and in the pool, about the dangers of alcohol and substance, which I had chosen to ignore for so many years because I was young and beautiful and having too much fun, came roaring back into my consciousness. So did fear about the damage I had already caused my body, and a desperation to arrest it as quickly as possible.

That was all it took. Overnight, I gave up the drinking and the drugs.

People find this story deeply dissatisfying – it is missing the rehab punchline, the inspiring arc of how I fought my way out of the abyss of addiction. What about the cold turkey, they ask me, the slow and painful process of withdrawal? Where is the hero's journey?

I don't know. Maybe it was 'sportsman's hangover' – the subliminal low that sportspeople experience when they are not in control of their bodies – that helped me walk away without a backward glance. Maybe it was the fact that I had taken to drinking merely to fully savour every aspect of the exciting new world that I had stumbled into and not as an escape from some unacknowledged trauma.

Or maybe the real reason, as I have now come to believe, after years of taking on and completing feats of endurance, is that the body's so-called needs, impulses and frailties are really those of the mind; if we are able to control the latter, the former will quietly, meekly, fall in line.

'Desire comes in waves. If you don't indulge it as soon as it rises in the mind, it will eventually fall – that is the nature of a wave. Once you realize that, you can control the desires you wish to.'

Sadly, quitting the drink and the drugs is not the end of my addiction story. A couple of years later, I fell into another one – smoking.

As if the steep highs, both literal and figurative, of the modelling years weren't enough, 1995 brought me even more attention, comprising in equal parts fame and notoriety, via a monster hit music video – for Alisha Chinai's peppy song, 'Made in India', in which I stepped topless out of a wooden crate and straight into the fantasies of Indian women everywhere; a controversial print ad for Tuff shoes, in which my then girlfriend, Madhu Sapre, and I were photographed in a clinch, wearing the shoes and a live python, but little else; and a pathbreaking television series, the first Indian series in English, called *A Mouthful of Sky*.

Shooting for television was very different from being on the modelling circuit, which was far more relaxed. *Mouthful* was a daily soap, so we shot 20 days a month, cooped up inside a studio for several hours a day. The cast was made up almost entirely of models like me, and many of them smoked to pass the time between takes. Ciggies being passed around was so much part of the culture of theatre, film sets and television studios in those days that you could fool yourself into believing it was a harmless bonding activity. By the time I first thought about quitting in 2001, I was smoking thirty cigarettes a day. What can I say? I am obsessive by nature.

Mouthful ran for a whole year. I was part of other serials after that, including the iconic *Captain Vyom*, in which I played the eponymous character, a courageous intergalactic superhero from India. There were a few Bollywood films as well, including, in 2002, the critically acclaimed *Agni Varsha* and *16 December*. I even turned film producer in that period, and cast myself as the romantic lead in a moderately successful film called *Rules: Pyaar ka Superhit Formula*.

Film sets were even more conducive to indulging a smoking habit – all one did for large parts of the day on film sets was wait for one's take to be called. Cigarettes and chai (another horrible habit I picked up during those years) were often an actor's only defence against mind-numbing boredom.

I might have continued forever along this path if someone hadn't mentioned, in passing, that international sports management company Procam was bringing to Bombay, in January 2004, India's very first professionally organized marathon, on the lines of the legendary Boston, New York and London marathons. My ears perked up. Deep inside my sportsman's heart, memories stretched and woke. Here, after a very long time, was the kind of challenge I had once thrived on, inviting me, enticing me, to bring my best physical, mental and emotional self to a feat of endurance. Suddenly, the thought of being inside a studio was anathema.

I wanted to be outside, on the streets, among the hills, inside the water, wild and free, one with the elements, my heart pumping, my limbs aching, honest sweat pouring down my face.

Moments later, other, less happy thoughts began to kick in. It was true I had been a champion once, but I was now 37, and had spent the last 15 years abusing my body with drink, drugs and nicotine. Would it now be up to a physical challenge, especially one that involved running, which I had never liked, let alone trained in? Was it even fair of me to expect it to?

There was only one way to find out what my body was capable of at 37, and that was to take on the challenge. So I did.

'Strive consistently to create new and challenging experiences for yourself. They will teach you more about you than anything else.'

For most of us, our life experiences are dictated not so much by us as by our circumstances and conditioning. We are sent to school, from where we move on to college and the workplace, acquiring a spouse and possibly children along the way, until, at the age of 60, we are told that we are no longer fit to work, and must now retire. This kind of arc necessarily means that our experiences are limited. How, then, can we know how we will cope with high-stress situations that fall outside our experience?

Simple. You must wilfully create new experiences for yourself, at every opportunity.

Thinking back, that was probably the reason I decided to run a half marathon at 37, 15 years after I had quit competitive sport. I had always detested running, even those laps around the pool that my coach used to make me do as a boy, and I wanted to understand if it came from a mental block or if there was something I really did not like about it. (I discovered it was the former.)

At 50, I attempted the Iron Man Triathlon, volunteering to put myself through another uniquely twisted form of torture, long-distance cycling. By now, I knew that I enjoyed setting myself challenges, and I wanted to see how my body and mind would react to the triathlon kind of challenge at my age.

I began to run barefoot for the same reason – a new experience. The theory that it is the most natural way to run appealed to me, and I wanted to try it for myself. It was difficult in the beginning, of course, but the human body is brilliant at adapting to new situations, and I soon began to appreciate the joy of moving in a way that connected me with the earth, where the feet communicated with the terrain at every step and adapted to it in real time.

A few years ago, I designed myself a new hat – motivational speaker. Why? Because I am essentially a shy person, who used to find it very difficult to speak to a large group of people. When people began to offer me money to do it, and it seemed that I could add value to other people's journeys in fitness by sharing my own, I decided the time had come to throw myself into this particular discomfort zone. The happiest spin-off of this has been the discovery that speaking about health and fitness clarifies things in my head, and helps me understand anew why fitness is important to me, and why I spend my days the way I do. Overall, this new career has been enormously self-validating. That validation brings me peace and gives me the impetus to keep going.

Not every new experience I seek ends in triumph and success. I wanted to include bugs and worms in my diet because I really believe they are the protein sources that can replace meat in human diets, thus arresting climate change, but broke out in a bad rash when I ate silkworms for the first time – turns out I'm allergic to chitin, the material that the exoskeleton of insects is made of. I cannot eat shellfish and scorpions for the same reason (I know because I tried them).

I haven't been able to learn to play a musical instrument or get over my fear of bungee jumping.

That does not stop me from trying new experiences, however, for the goal is clear – it isn't to succeed at everything I try but to increase my level of self-awareness. I push myself into uncomfortable situations because I find it incredibly interesting to see what comes up – in my mind, in my body – when I am in them. It is the journey from discomfort to comfort that I find fascinating because it has taught me, over and over, that the situation is never the problem, it's me.

The moment I had made the decision to sign up for the half marathon, I knew exactly what I had to do. For the next few months, until Race Day, I would have to go back to eating fresh, wholesome food, at regular mealtimes. I would have to cut out the late-night parties to ensure that I would be in bed early and out at dawn, pounding the streets. I would have to take on less television and film work to be able to create the time and mindspace required for this demanding new passion project. Most importantly, since this challenge would require my lungs to be in their best possible shape, the cigarettes would have to go.

I had realized that I was sliding down a very slippery slope with the cigarettes a couple of years earlier. But I hadn't reckoned with the addictive nature of nicotine. No matter how hard I tried, I found myself unable to kick the habit. Now, finally, I had found both the incentive and the impetus to clean up my act.

As for the actual mechanics of quitting, I came up with something as disarmingly simple in theory as it turned out to be in practice – procrastination. Whenever I felt like a cigarette, I told myself I would have one in ten minutes, and got busy doing something else. By the time ten minutes had passed, the desire had passed too. That was really it!

'If you have to have an addiction, pick one that's good for you.'

People are incredulous when I tell them my patented method for quitting a bad habit. I suppose it is only fair, therefore, that I tell you the rest of my quitting story. Whether with alcohol or cigarettes, I had almost always indulged in the free stuff, which ensured that I never drank or smoked alone. With cigarettes, particularly, I had never bought one, preferring to bum one off a friend or a co-star

– that was a big part of the excitement of going to the sets. There was an element of self-deception involved – if I didn't buy fags, I told myself, I wasn't really addicted to the stuff. Plus, smoking was just something I did at the workplace. There was no question of doing it at home, in any case – if there was anything Aai detested more than alcohol, it was cigarettes. Essentially, there was work involved in finding a cigarette – I could not mindlessly reach for another one. Perhaps that helped in the quitting process.

Thinking back, I wonder why the temptation to buy a pack never overcame me. It certainly wasn't because I could not afford it. However, in another sense, somewhere deep down, I suppose I knew that I could not afford it at all.

Can we afford 'festival food' every day? Many of us can – Indian sweets and namkeen cost a fraction of what good chocolate does. But can we really, in another sense, *afford* it? Can our bodies take the burden of the large amounts of fat and sugar such foods contain, on a daily or even weekly basis? Is it fair to expect our physiological systems not to protest, break down, give up, when we abuse them that way?

Surely not. Why do we do it then? And then, when our health begins to fail or we decide we do not 'look good', why do we rush in the opposite direction, abusing our bodies in a different way with diets that may not be good for us? Why do we overdo the exercise routines with a short-term, short-sighted weight loss goal in mind, instead of a long-term goal of good health?

Because our bodies are disconnected from our minds. Because we never ask ourselves the right questions. People approach me all the time, everywhere, to ask me for advice on what they should do to lose weight and become fit. When I ask them why they want to lose weight, the answers, from both men and women, are almost always the same. 'I am getting married in two months and want to look good in the photographs'; 'I am in the market for a partner and want to be able to attract the best ones'; 'I want to fit into the clothes in my closet.' When I ask them why they want to be fit, they are usually confounded, until they say, with a somewhat puzzled expression, 'Because . . . it's good to be fit, no?'

What these answers tell me is that neither group is thinking for themselves, or indeed, of themselves, even though they believe they are. If I was asked why I take care of myself in the ways I do, I have only one answer – 'Because I love being able to do the things I am doing, and would like to continue doing them. Because I want to avoid being sick, as far as possible. Because I want to make sure everything is working. To achieve that, I need to drive the vehicle of the body in such a way that the battery does not run down. I need to use the right fuel to power it, and I need to take it for a spin each day, to ensure it is running smoothly.' That kind of answer makes both logical and emotional sense to me. It makes me reach for an apple instead of a piece of chocolate when both options are available, without wasting a moment's thought on the decision.

If my answers sound to you like the right answers, what are the right questions? Ask yourself – 'WHAT do I want for myself in this life? WHY do I want it?' The questions sound simple enough, but answering them will require deep introspection. Here's a useful tip: make sure your answers make both logical and emotional sense to you. If they only make logical sense – you understand why you want to do it in your head, but not in your heart – the goals will not find as deep a resonance. If they only make emotional sense – you *feel* very strongly about them, but can't explain why they are important – you will not be able to sustain the lifestyle required to achieve your goals. Especially once your immediate motivation, like looking good in a wedding photograph, has passed.

If you define your goals clearly, however, you will automatically, almost unconsciously, begin to do things that align with them. That's the only trick there is.

'Clear thinking' is seldom cited as the foundation of a physically healthy life, but it is vital. It is our thoughts that power our choices – simply put, we become what we think. If we let our choices be powered by our 'feelings', it means that we have stopped thinking, and that is never a good thing.

Do I regret abusing my body during the 15 years that I spent away from active sport? Not at all – regret is a complete waste of time and energy. Every experience we live through changes us in some way, but it is how we remember those experiences and how we assimilate and make sense of them – all of which is in our control – that decide whether we are changed positively or negatively. It was through the experiences of those years that I came to understand myself much better than I had ever before. I realized, for instance, that I had an addictive personality. That knowledge helped me tremendously – if I could not help being addicted, I would actively choose things that were good for me to get addicted to.

I chose running that long ago day in 2003, and I chose to prioritize the outdoors over the studios. To this day, I have remained happily addicted to both.

LET'S GO! HOW TO BEGIN YOUR OWN FITNESS JOURNEY

1. **Start with a minute.** Do just *one minute* of exercise, any exercise. Every single day. When you feel comfortable in the routine, up it to two minutes, then five.

2. **Experiment with food.** Choose one specific grain, any grain, and eat just that for a week. See how it makes your body feel. Try a different one the next week. Understand what food makes your body comfortable.

3. **Increase your good habits, decrease your bad habits.** You know what your bad food and fitness habits are. Every day, do them a little less.

4. **Go to bed around the same time each day.** A fixed sleep schedule will train your body and mind to expect it, and prep for it.

5. **Bring your body back to its childlike state.** Take the stairs down two at a time, leap up to touch a tree branch, swing from the hanging roots of a banyan. For the joy of it.

THE THING ABOUT MILIND

Milind has an unusual mind – I may not always agree with him but I admire how his mind works. I wonder often where he inherited it from – not from me or my husband, for sure. He is a very independent thinker – he develops his own philosophy, whether it is about life, food, fitness, relationships, science, religion or anything else, and doesn't follow anyone. He is very persuasive as well – no one can argue with his ideas, however unconventional. I tell him he should have been a lawyer.

He isn't very rigid about things, not even exercise or diet – he loves khichdi and can eat it every day, but he doesn't fuss if there's something else on the table. He did overdo things for a brief period when he was younger, but not anymore – he may have a drink occasionally, in company, but he is happy without as well.

I feel compelled to add, for the benefit of people who may only know of him for the last couple of decades, that he never used to dress like this before, wearing the same two T-shirts and trackpants day after day – he used to be a fashion icon.

– Usha

I admire Milind's discipline and the level of activity he is able to sustain through the day. He simply does not know how to rest. He very rarely takes responsibility for things, but once he does, you can be sure that the task will be done to perfection. He is affected very little by things that are happening around him (which can be annoying for people), but his emotional health is excellent because of this ability. He never blindly follows trends – he will question everything, do his research and come up with his own conclusion about whether there is any useful takeaway from it or not. If there isn't, he will drop it without a second thought. He is logical and balanced – I'm not always so, and that's why I admire those qualities and rely on them so much.

– Ankita

ANKITA

From Light to Darkness and Back to Light

'Life makes no promises. What is the guarantee that you and your love will grow old together? Instead of focusing on the future, enjoy every moment.'

K came into my life when he and I were 16, in a pair of bright yellow shoes. By then, I had finished my tenth grade and moved to the B. Borooah College in Guwahati for my higher secondary (the equivalent of Grades 11 and 12). In a very uncharacteristic move – I usually keep to myself around people, and avoid the spotlight as much as possible – I walked up to him to ask him about his flashy shoes. In that first conversation, a deep connection was established. We became instantly inseparable, bonding as classmates, friends and soulmates. He was far more sophisticated than I in terms of his exposure – his dad worked in oil, and so he had lived around the country, and even in the Gulf for a bit – and I was in awe of that. He was also passionate about bikes, which made him cool in my eyes.

I was never in the habit of keeping things that brought me happiness from my parents, so they were in the know about my boyfriend right from the beginning, as was Maina.

Like any pair of high school sweethearts, K and I planned our future together. He loved travelling and so did I, so we decided to get our BSc degrees in Hospitality Management and Tourism from a professional institute after higher secondary.

My family is full of people who studied science and went on to become teachers and academics, or people who worked for the government. The things I wanted were very different, but there was no one to guide me as to what courses to take. So I took my own decisions, as always. One of the reasons I chose to do the BSc I did was that I knew I would be employable at the end of it. I was good at oral and written communication, and was confident of landing a job in the campus recruitment week itself.

I was also very keen on English – I nurtured, and still do, dreams of being a writer – so I applied and got into the BA (English) undergrad programme at my old college B. Borooah as well. It was quite a crazy decision – it meant juggling attendance requirements at both courses and commuting between campuses each day, but I was happy to be working towards what I wanted.

Our lives were set. K and I were full of hope and confidence that the world of glamorous hotels, airports and exotic international destinations would be our oyster. In any case, Putha, who had astrology as one of his side hustles, had read my palm and told me I would travel a lot around the world. In the selective way in which we all take such information, I had embraced this bit because it fit so nicely with my own dream and ignored some of the other things Putha had read in my palm, including that I would marry a man very much older than I.

I was hugely inspired by the financially independent teenagers I saw in American sitcoms, and did not want to bother my parents for money. For pocket money, therefore, K and I took on small jobs wherever and whenever we could. We might be handing out pamphlets at a street corner or ushering people into auditoriums or helping at music events or art exhibitions, but we always had money of our own for little luxuries and treats, a wonderful thing when you're at college.

Despite K and I being such an 'item', however, I continued to be very much my own person, still spending a lot of time by myself, although, in Guwahati, I walked more and cycled less. Borooah College is quite close to Pan Bazaar, and I usually set off from there at some point in the early evening, headphones in place. I would turn around only when I was absolutely forced to, at Khanapara, which is at Assam's border with Meghalaya. The whole loop was close to 20 kilometres, but I didn't think at all about the distance then. **To me, the walks were about precious, purposeless me-time, which I valued immensely.**

In my second year of college, Papa got transferred to Guwahati. After many, many years of looking out for myself, I had a best friend (who was also my boyfriend) to share my dreams with, and my family to return to each evening. It was the best of times.

Until that phone call.

Every year, around February, IIT Guwahati hosts their iconic three-day inter-collegiate cultural festival, Alcheringa, the largest of its kind in the Northeast. Like every other young person in Guwahati, K and I were there, mostly to check out the bands and their music. You can imagine what the atmosphere was like – the air was thick with banned substances and most people were as high as kites.

But we hadn't gone there together. The previous evening, we had got into an ugly spat about something that now seems inconsequential. I was furious, perhaps disproportionately so. I had said a lot of things to him that I will forever be sorry about, to which he had responded with equally mean words. It had ended with me telling him to 'go to hell' and walking off.

When K found out from one of his friends that I was at Alcheringa, he began calling and texting me repeatedly. I suppose he wanted to apologize and make up, so that we could enjoy the festival together. But I was still hurting, so I did not respond.

The next morning, feeling bad about my behaviour, I began making his favourite kheer and poori, wondering why he hadn't picked up my calls inviting him to lunch. When he did not call back by mid-morning, I began to get a little concerned and called a friend who had been with him the previous evening. There was a long silence at the other end of the line, before the friend, his voice breaking, gave me the news. After I had left in anger and not taken his calls, K had gotten very agitated. When he decided to leave the festival, still very upset, he had given his bike to a friend to drive him home – he *never* did that, he loved his bike too much to trust anyone else with it – and ridden pillion without a helmet.

The truck had come out of nowhere. When it had raced away, there was very little left of K. I never got to say goodbye because no one would let me see his mangled body. He was only 20.

'Trauma teaches you a lot about yourself, helps you become your own best friend. You have to believe that you have what it takes to climb out of the dark hole – because you do.'

My world went dark. For months after, the grief was so overwhelming that there was only one thought hammering away in my head – I want to die, I want to die. In my own amateurish way, I tried more than once to kill myself – it seemed the 'right' thing to do, for then, as I told myself, my pain would be at an end, and my parents would not have to lose sleep over me anymore. Once, I overdosed on sleeping pills and had to be rushed to the hospital. Another time, I slit my wrists, but was 'found out' in time and rescued. Perhaps, subconsciously, I prevented myself from going all the way – not because of a hardwired self-preservation instinct, but because each time I decided to try something like this, Papa's face would enter my head, unbidden. Looking back now, I see that even when I had reached rock bottom, my predominant concern was that I should not cause my parents trouble – just the thought of how devastated Papa would be if I took my life was enough to stay in my hand.

I realized with a sinking heart that there was going to be no quick, easy way out of my suffering. The suicidal thoughts

I had been feeling were replaced with a blank, paralysing numbness.

My life stretched before me endlessly – dull, hopeless, devoid of goals, dreams and purpose. My long-cherished desire of going to France for my master's degree now seemed utterly pointless. I had nothing to share or discuss with people of my own age, who were consumed, as K and I had been, with long-term career and relationship goals. I went through the motions of what was left of college life like an automaton, and spent hours and hours sitting in my balcony, staring at nothing, or going back to the place where the accident had happened and howling, inundated with guilt and remorse for my parting words to him. I knew I was making my parents sick with worry, but I was helpless, unable to rouse myself from my desolation to become even a shadow of their cheerful little girl again.

It was Maina who sent out job applications in my name after I'd graduated and forced me to attend interviews. Convinced that what I needed was a radical change of scene, she had sent in an application to a Malaysia-based airline called AirAsia that was looking to enter India in a few months' time. When I received the interview call, she forced me to clean up nice, checked that my clothes were presentable and dropped me to the hotel where the interview was taking place, not trusting that I would actually attend it otherwise. I walked in and took my place in line, and was informed that should I get picked, the training would happen in Kuala Lumpur.

I had paid little attention to the company that was doing the hiring until then, but with that piece of information, something shifted. Deep inside, a tiny spark of the old wanderlust came alive. I aced the interview. In May 2013, just a few months before my twenty-second birthday, I was winging my way to Malaysia to begin a new life.

'Just like the good times, the tough times do not last. The trick lies in staying afloat long enough to outlast them.'

But simply swapping one outer world for another never really helps with flushing out the murky, viscous stuff that roils our inner worlds, does it? The darkness, and the numbness, followed me to Malaysia. I was doing very well at work, learning quickly, being noticed by my seniors. I had work colleagues that I vibed well with. I was earning more money than I ever had. I still walked when I could – to the mall, to restaurants, anywhere I needed to go that was within a 5 kilometre radius. When the training was done and I started flying as part of the cabin crew, I got to stay at the best hotels and eat lavishly.

I went from buffet to lavish buffet in a sleep-deprived haze, indiscriminately eating sugar-laden, fat-heavy foods, anything that gave my palate instant gratification, telling myself I needed it or, worse, *deserved* it for all the hard work I was putting in, all the while looking for something that could make me feel less dead inside. At 22, I was a disaster waiting to happen.

Pretty soon, the explosive cocktail of youth, emptiness, money, access and peer pressure ensured that I was on the slippery slope to addiction. The culture allowed it, even encouraged it. Party as hard as you like, as long as you also work as hard, seemed to be the unspoken rule. I embraced it wholeheartedly. Tobacco, alcohol and other substances became part of my daily diet – I chased the highs and the oblivion they afforded, for anything, *anything*, was better than the relentless pain.

It was the worst of times.

In early 2014, the first batch of AirAsia's cabin crew moved back to India, to Chennai, the first India headquarters of the airline. The first domestic flight was scheduled to take off in April or May, and as the pressure of work got higher, so did the partying. One night, as I was dancing and drinking myself silly, as per usual, in the nightclub of the hotel where we were staying, I noticed the atmosphere in the room had suddenly turned electric. Looking around, I saw why – Captain Vyom was in the houuuuuuuse!

I had grown up watching the amazing adventures of the home-grown intergalactic superhero, Captain Vyom, on Doordarshan, and had been thrilled to catch sight of him – more correctly, the actor who played him, but in my mind the two were inseparable – in the hotel over the last two days. I had dearly wanted to go up and say hello but hadn't because I did not want to bother him. Now he was in the same room as I, relaxed, dancing, having a good time. If I didn't say hello now, I never would. With my friends pushing me forward, I went up to him and told him how much I had enjoyed Captain Vyom. He asked me to dance with him, and I did, thrilled. A couple of songs later, I told him I was stepping out for a smoke and left, feeling wonderful to have met and interacted with a childhood hero, but nothing else.

I certainly did not dream that Captain Vyom would ask my friends for my number after I'd gone. Or that he would be the one to help me climb out of the deep dark pit I had fallen into and give myself another chance at love and life.

If there's one truth I've come to believe in implicitly in my admittedly short life, it is this: 'Nothing goes according to plan. Life is flow. Your best bet is to flow with it.'

'The only way through pain is gratitude. Intervention by others can help, but only in a limited way. In the end, only you have the power to heal yourself.'

Milind and I began seeing each other very soon after that night in the club. To everyone else, it seemed like a most unlikely pairing, doomed to failure, especially given my extreme youth (I was still 22) and the difference in our ages (he is 26 years older) but to the two of us, it felt right from the word go. I was still hurting too much from K's loss to look at anyone else around my own age as a potential partner, so the age difference turned out to be an advantage as far as I was concerned.

I have no idea why Milind felt I was right for him among all the other women clamouring for his attention, but I can tell you why he was right for me. He was exactly what I needed at that fragile, vulnerable stage in my life – a beautiful, sorted, secure man who had nothing left to prove.

He cared deeply about me and loved the same things I did – family, nature, travel, physical activity, me-time. We shared the same philosophical bent of mind, we were each of us essentially self-sufficient, emotionally speaking (well, I wasn't, not at the time, but you know what I mean), and we both loved to eat.

Most importantly, he did not flinch once at my dark side, which he saw a lot of in the first two to three years of our relationship. Instead, he supported me lovingly and patiently through my episodes. Once, in 2015, overwhelmed by a sudden flood of sadness, I went up to the tenth floor of the apartment building in Gurgaon where I was living alone at the time, determined to throw myself off it. Once again, remembering Papa saved me. When I told Milind about it, he simply listened calmly and held me close. A less emotionally secure person would have made it about himself, feeling hurt or getting mad that all the love he had poured into me had not been enough to turn suicidal thoughts from my head. Not Milind.

But I still resisted committing to him for the longest time, because, as I told him, I still felt very committed to K, and it didn't seem fair that he, Milind, would never have my entire heart as a result. His response won me over. 'He was part of you when I met you,' he said. 'Why would I want you to lose a part of yourself to become mine? You don't have to let go of him, ever.'

When I met him, Milind Soman was already a huge inspiration to women across the country. Since 2012, his company had organized all-women running events around the country under the brand name Pinkathon, through which he exhorted women to put themselves and their health front and centre (in fact, the reason he was at the hotel where I met him was that Chennai's very first Pinkathon was happening a few days later). In 2014, he also became mine (my inspiration, I mean, but also, just mine).

But it wasn't just Milind who helped me begin the process of healing – it was also his entire family. Aai, who had always got along with any girl Milind had dated, accepted me just as easily. So did his sisters, his brothers-in-law, and his nephews and nieces. That kind of unquestioning, loving acceptance is not easy to come by for an odd couple – I mean, my mum is younger than Milind, and I am younger than a couple of his nephews – in any family, Indian or otherwise! We would only marry in 2018, but they treated me like one of them right from the start. With this whole new family supporting me, how could I not want to be the best version of myself?

Even so, it would take time for me to truly begin to love myself enough again. When I turned 25, I decided the time had come to begin making the small lifestyle changes. For starters, I began eating more mindfully. This was a tough one, because food was always so plentifully available around me, whether in the hotels the cabin crew stayed at or in the air. But slowly and surely, I nixed the chocolate bars and ice tea that were my standard inflight sustenance and brought my own snacks from home instead – usually, a simple, protein-rich salad involving sprouts or kala chana. Looking back, I realize I had never really enjoyed the chocolate bars or the ice tea that much – I had reached for them simply because they were there.

In any case, most 22-year-olds who have led a reasonably active life and eaten reasonably healthy food have such good metabolism that they can usually eat and digest anything without tangible consequences. The moment I began to think about what I was eating, however, the easy titbits, empty of nutrition, lost their appeal. Plus, **switching up my daily snack made a big difference to my own sense of well-being – I was actively choosing to eat better, which made me feel virtuous, responsible and most importantly, in control.**

That made me a happier person, and that happiness changed the energy around me in many little ways. I began having actual conversations with passengers on my flights, and they responded with equal warmth, some of them mentioning me by name in mails of appreciation they sent to the airline. I began to feel more positive, more hopeful, less burdened by the darkness. I began to actively look forward to each day, feeling light and young and carefree again.

I'm not sure **which comes first in a virtuous cycle – do you feel grateful because you are happy, or does happiness come out of an innate sense of gratitude for what you have?** Who knows. I suppose that's why it is called a cycle – how do you tell where a cycle begins and where it ends? Whatever. The thing was this: by and by, I found gratitude in my life again. I felt deep appreciation for my body, which had taken such abuse without foundering. I felt a huge sense of thankfulness for the partner I had found, my job, the childhood my parents and grandparents had given me, for my darling sister. I felt blessed to be even breathing, to be still standing when others around me had been cut down in the prime of their youth. I began to gingerly revisit the memories I had locked away in the deepest recesses of my mind and taught myself to cherish them, to be thankful that they had happened at all instead of feeling devastated that the people who helped make them were gone.

It was a slow, slow process, with many setbacks, but it felt so good to be moving forward, even if it was only by inches, that I felt compelled to persist. And for that, once again, I am grateful.

THE THING ABOUT ANKITA

What I admire about Ankita is her determination and her competitive streak – if she decides she wants to achieve some goal, she will do it. She didn't run very much at all before she met Milind, but she decided to begin doing what he enjoys and now she runs marathons! She is very conversant, like others of her generation, with digital media – very sharp, very quick. What I also like about her is that she will eat anything she is served. She cleans her plate. No fuss at all. She loves her meat, especially pork, and will eat very well if it is on the table.

– Usha

Ankita is a very quick learner. She takes a long time to decide that she wants to learn something, but once she has made up her mind, she learns quickly and well. She had never learnt to swim, but when we were in the Maldives, she met an Italian girl who persuaded her to go scuba diving with her. That got her over her fear of water. In 2023 the urge to compete in the Iron Man Triathlon took over her mind. You can't do a triathlon without knowing how to swim, and so she started swimming lessons. Just two months later, she swam a kilometre!

– Milind

THE SOMAN SUTRA: THE BEST EXERCISE FOR A FIT BODY

Usha: Walking! You don't need equipment – no mat, no shoes, no props, no costume. You don't need a trainer or a coach. You don't need to warm up or warm down. There isn't even a right way to do it. Just get up and walk, any time! Walk briskly outside the house, not inside, every day if possible, for at least 15 minutes. Don't use your walk time to catch up with a friend on the phone or listen to music – instead, have an uninterrupted conversation with yourself.

Milind: Running brings a lot of joy, but it is the most inefficient exercise. In terms of efficiency, few exercises can beat this most natural one: Sit on the floor and get up without using your hands, all in one fluid motion. To do this well, you will need to have opened your hips, opened your knees, and developed core strength. Do this for three minutes each day, with some variations thrown in, and you are fit!

Ankita: Suryanamaskar and running. The first is amazing for building strength and mobility, the second is excellent for the heart and for building endurance. Exercise every day – unless you are a pro athlete, you don't need a rest day. Thirty minutes a day of exercise is more than enough for anyone, but if you can only take 15 minutes out, do it, and make sure you are 100% present. Mindfulness during exercise is more important than the routine itself.

THE SOMAN SUTRA: THE BEST TOOL TO FIGHT LAZY

Usha: Discipline. Tell your mind that you simply have to do whatever you had planned to do, and don't allow it to make any excuses.

Milind: To make your mind your ally instead of your adversary, get your priorities straight. If you've planned a 6 a.m. run, and you've been invited to a party the night before that starts at 10 p.m., you can't do both. Ask yourself which is more important, and stick to your choice. Make decisions easy for your mind, by reducing them to simple, logical yes/no questions.

Ankita: Bargain with yourself on the days when all you want to do is stay in bed. I coax myself out of lethargy by saying things like, 'Just do six suryanamaskars, not the twelve you had planned. Okay fine, do three . . .' That makes it easier for me to begin, and usually, once I begin, I end up doing all twelve. Never, ever give yourself the option of skipping the routine entirely.

THE SOMAN SUTRA:
WHY GYMS DON'T CUT IT (FOR ME)

Usha: Gyms? Never been inside one, mostly because I haven't been able to understand the appeal of going indoors to exercise.

Milind: I don't need the machines, I don't need the mirrors and I like being outdoors. Historically, gyms were built for pro athletes and bodybuilders, and for physiotherapy and rehab, not for general fitness. It is the community-building factor that gyms capitalize on today to draw people in. If you don't need the community, and you are more into fitness than bodybuilding, you don't need a gym.

Ankita: Ummm, honestly? I don't like how they smell (sorry!), and I find them a little claustrophobic. Other reasons? It feels very competitive and the routines feel generic, not customized to me. Also, the sight of other people working out distracts me from my practice – I find myself judging people or feeling judged by them. Either way, I lose the focus that is so vital to any fitness practice.

SECTION 3

STAYING THE COURSE

For Every Reason, in Every Season

When does the delight in the new and exciting turn into the tiresome slog of the mundane? Very quickly, for our monkey minds, forever engaged in their quest for novelty and distraction, are incredibly difficult to restrain. Yet – and this is common, lived knowledge – it is only by following the discipline of doing a thing over and over again that, organically, almost unconsciously, you gain mastery of that thing. Call it habit or muscle memory, but once it is built, that mastery is incredibly difficult to lose. That is why it is so important to be mindful each day of the things we choose – and it is always a choice – to do over and over. How we live our days – staying active (or not), eating right (or not), jettisoning negativity (or not), nurturing a grateful heart (or not) – is how we live our lives.

USHA

Growing Old in the Body Is Inevitable – Growing Old in the Mind, Inexcusable

'I took my first purposeless walk at the age of 57. I had just retired, and was bored, so I decided to try this "walking" fad. Until then, my life had only been full of purposeful walking.'

Throughout my life, I have walked everywhere – to school, to the market, to buy groceries, to the bank, to pay electricity and telephone bills, to buy train tickets . . . Today, people don't even need to move out of their beds to do these things. In addition, they are all eating ready-to-eat food. Packaged food is convenient, for sure, but it is also processed, and as consumers, we have no idea how that processing affects our digestive systems in the long run. There is a list of ingredients on the package, but a lot of them are chemicals that we as consumers know nothing about.

It's a bit of a tragedy as I see it, not just because of the damage processed food may cause, but because not cooking your own food also means missing the joy of being among fresh produce, choosing what you will cook based on what vegetable or bunch of greens looks freshest, picking through heaps of fruit while letting your eyes, nose, tongue and fingers be the judges of what comes home to the family and then lovingly turning all of it into food that everyone enjoys. The modern age has brought so many blessings, but the lifestyle is detrimental to individual and societal health – there's a loss of human connection, as I mentioned earlier, a paralysing dependence on devices and apps, and the danger of eating without awareness or gratitude of what is on your plate because you did not spend time and effort over making it.

But enough with the angsty detour. Back to my story. I used to drive in England, but I never did in India. (Milind and Ankita both have their drivers' licences, but they don't drive either.) Bombay has always had great public transport, so I have never missed having my own vehicle. Once the children were settled and I started working in the biochemistry department of Wilson College, I walked, every working day for several years, from home to Dadar station. It took me about 15 minutes on a good day, 12 if I was running late. From there, I took the local to Charni Road and then walked from the station to college, a similar distance. On the way back, I repeated the whole thing in reverse. Even at work, since I was in charge of the biochemistry lab, I was on my feet a lot.

When I retired from college, there was suddenly nothing to do. My husband had passed three years previously, of a heart attack; he had had his first one back in England, but the second one, which he suffered when he was only 63, proved to be fatal. The children were all grown – my youngest, Anupama, was herself over 30 – and, apart from Milind, had moved out of home. Others of my age had long succumbed to the seductions of television as an evening 'activity', but I wasn't habituated to it – in all the years since the early '70s when Doordarshan started broadcasting to Bombay, we had never bought a television; my husband did not care for it. It was Milind who finally bought me a television in 1995, so that I could watch him on TV. He had just started his television career as one of the leads in *A Mouthful Of Sky*. The novelist Ashok Banker had written the script for it, and it aired every weekday – they shot over 250 episodes!

But to go back to my retirement. Reading and the radio kept me happily occupied for part of the day, and there was always some housework, but the discovery that there were now very few opportunities for me to be unthinkingly, casually, active horrified me.

That was when I started walking with no purpose – three rounds of Shivaji Park each morning, simply to feel the joy of moving briskly. It was freeing to be able to walk without having to watch the clock – I did not have anywhere to get to by a particular time. That habit, which I adopted no sooner than I retired and have kept up for the last 24 years, is what has kept me so limber. **I truly believe in the power of keeping your body moving. Resting too much will only cause your muscles to atrophy and your joints to get rusty. It's not rocket science; it's common sense.**

I'm glad that people have understood this, and wilful 'exercise' has become part of many of their lives. But I am not in favour of the way it is marketed – almost as if it were a chore one has been compelled to do (because, if it wasn't a chore, why would anyone need a 'cheat day' or a 'taking it easy day' as a reward for their commitment?). I do not agree with the concept of doing so many 'reps' of a routine for so many hours, so that you can look or feel a certain way. I think the whole preoccupation with six packs and sculpted bodies is unhealthy and show-off-y, meant more to elicit the envy of others than to cultivate good health for oneself. It all gets very competitive, and competition is a huge stress;

it takes a toll on your mental health, which reflects in your physical health.

This is one of the reasons why I liked the concept of Pinkathon so much, the women's running event that Milind's company, Maximus, launched in Mumbai 2012. It was all about joy – the joy of so many women together, owning the space around them for a few hours, the joy of being away from one's responsibilities and duties and doing something solely for oneself, which women so rarely allow themselves, the joy of moving free and unfettered in their T-shirts and tracks and salwars and even sarees, without having to wonder if they were looking 'decent' – the joy, really, of being themselves. The way women responded to the event was incredible – again and again I heard them tell Milind, 'We haven't run since high school! Thank you for giving us this opportunity!'

The very next year, Maximus got the opportunity to help Oxfam organize their first Trailwalker in Mumbai. The Trailwalker is a walking event in which people participate as teams of four, not as individuals. You can choose to do either the 50 kilometre walk, which is to be completed within 24 hours, or the 100 kilometre one, which is to be completed within 48 hours. The route of the walk is designed to take participants through some lovely, picturesque countryside. Encouraged and inspired by Pinkathon energy, my daughters and I decided to participate in the Trailwalker as a team, just for the heck of it. We chose the 100 kilometre walk for a lark, fully prepared to not complete it. But to our own surprise, we did! In 41 hours! It was such a lovely, family-bonding experience – we enjoyed it so very much. And so we did the Trailwalker again in 2014, and then again in 2015, when I was 76.

I felt invincible, unstoppable. I had never done push-ups or planks in my life before, but when Milind asked me to try, I did, and found that I could. In 2016, a video of me running barefoot in a saree on a highway, alongside Milind, went viral. There was nothing planned about that – it was entirely happenstance. Milind was running from Ahmedabad to Mumbai at the time, and I was waiting at the point where he would enter Maharashtra to welcome him and cheer him as he ran by. When he spotted me, he waved and asked me to join him for a bit, and I jumped in. It was cumbersome to run in the slippers I was wearing, so I kicked them off, hitched up my saree and ran. People thought that was something marvellous, but it never felt like I was doing anything extraordinary. It felt natural and normal, and not because running was something I did regularly either. I am used to getting up and moving when an occasion demands it, and this occasion demanded running, so that's what I did.

In 2018, my daughters and I did a different kind of long

walk, with Milind and Ankita, in a different country. The two of them had already been married in a traditional Assamese ceremony in Mumbai, but they also wanted to get married in a church. They picked the eleventh-century Cathedral of Santiago de Compostela in Spain, and decided to literally walk to their wedding, except the walk was 600 kilometres long! Starting from Lisbon, Portugal, they planned to walk along the ninth-century pilgrimage route called the Camino de Santiago, over 20 days. The rest of the family was invited to join in as well, and I agreed enthusiastically. Netra, Medha and Anupama demurred, saying they would join us just for the Spain leg of the Camino de Santiago. I must say that was a wonderful experience as well. On my eightieth birthday, I did 16 push-ups, which one of the children recorded on their phone and broadcast. That video also became very popular and was shared a lot.

In November 2020, when I was 81, I completed the 52 kilometre Sandakphu trek in West Bengal, with Milind and Ankita. I had always wanted to do the trek, and COVID presented the perfect opportunity. Milind's crazy travel schedule had come to a complete stop, and he was champing at the bit, wanting to get away. When he suggested Sandakphu, even though I knew it would be freezing in the mountains at that time of year, I agreed with alacrity. Over the course of the trek, we climbed from around 6,400 feet to almost 12,000 feet, and were rewarded at the top with a glorious sunset and spectacular views of Chomolungma (Mount Everest) and Khangchengdzonga (Kanchenjunga). Later, the Himalayan Mountaineering Institute informed us that, going by their records, I was the oldest woman to have ever done the trek. Can you imagine!

And all of this, *all* of this – the planks, the push-ups, the Trailwalker, Sandakphu – had become possible not because I had been 'in training' to do any of it, not because I regularly 'worked out' at a gym, but simply because I had never stopped moving. I think the fact that we as a family have always done sporty, outdoorsy things together is also very much part of this. It's not just the joy of moving, but also the joy of doing it with people you love.

Whenever young people, particularly young women, ask me for tips on staying healthy or fit, I think of Pinkathon. And this is the advice I give them: Take so much joy in movement, make it so much a part of your life that you would not take a rest day if it was offered to you on a platter – seriously, why would you want to sit in one place and do nothing when you have legs that can take you places? If you can't schedule time for the gym or a fitness routine, just walk to places instead of getting into a car – there really is no exercise as complete and beneficial as walking, if you do it every single day. Be mindful of your posture – keep your spine long and your back erect whether you are sitting, standing or walking, because that will keep your mind alert and your senses alive. (At 84, I have only lost an inch in height – I am now 5 feet 4 inches instead of 5 feet 5 inches, and I believe that is largely due to good posture.) **Most importantly, only compete with yourself each day, asking if you are a better person today than you were yesterday; if you moved more lightly, more easily, more compassionately.**

'I did not eat breakfast for many, many years of my life. Now I do, religiously. Your body's needs change with age and stage. Just listen to your body.'

When the children were young, the mornings were always very busy, with breakfast to be served and lunch to be kept ready for when they got back from school, since I was always at work at that time. Milind used to attend the afternoon shift at school; I remember he helped me a lot with the cooking in the mornings. Either way, I never had time to eat breakfast, so my system got used to it. I did not have breakfast for many, many years of my life.

I did not carry a lunchbox to college either, because I like to eat my food hot. In those days, there were very few restaurants around the college, and certainly none that I could casually pop into for a quick bite of lunch – women did not do things like that. It was only when I got home from college, around 2.30 in the afternoon, that I would settle down for my first meal of the day – a long, relaxed, hot lunch, all by myself. I savoured every morsel of my meal then, chewing slowly and deliberately, thinking of nothing but the food. That habit has persisted. My children and Ankita tease me about how very slowly I eat, but ask any doctor or philosopher, and they will tell you that it isn't just *what* we eat that makes us, but *how* we eat it.

Just before COVID hit, I had started developing varicose veins. The swelling around my ankles and feet had begun even before the Sandakphu trek, but I had never let on. With the world shutting down, we left Bombay and spent long periods in Milind's house in Lonavala, which made it difficult to have my condition seen to. I kept myself active and took care of my condition in ways that seemed right to me, because I really, really hate making a fuss. My threshold for pain is high, so no one around me realized there was anything wrong.

Also, with COVID thick in the air, it was inadvisable to go to a hospital, particularly because none of us – Milind, Ankita or I – had taken the COVID vaccine. Ankita and Milind did not take it because they contracted COVID before it was their turn to get the vaccine, and I – well, I did not take it because I did not want to.

Let me explain. I am a biochemist, my husband was a pharmacologist and my father-in-law had been director of the Haffkine Institute, so I understand something about vaccines. I found it very difficult to believe not only that a vaccine could be produced so quickly but also that it could be rigorously tested in so short a time. I preferred, therefore, to trust my immune system and nurture my body with nutritious food, instead of subjecting myself to the vaccine.

But my varicose veins got worse, and then the children began to worry. They fretted that I wasn't healing fast enough despite all the hot water I was steeping my legs in. They insisted I go and see a doctor. My only response, which I kept repeating to them, was, 'Don't tell me what to do, or I will lose my confidence. I know my limitations, and I will not overdo anything. Believe me when I tell you that my condition isn't hampering me – I would know better than you about that, wouldn't I?'

But that situation changed. Despite all the precautions I was taking, by August 2022, my condition deteriorated to the point where I was forced to go into hospital to have it attended to. Surgery was recommended. I came back home in a wheelchair.

It was a shock of cataclysmic proportions for me. After the highs, both literal and metaphorical, of Sandakphu, I had been brought down to earth with a bang. Not to be mobile in the way I was used to was a huge, huge setback. The children insisted I get a cook. I had no choice but to agree. The doctors said it would probably take me three months to begin walking comfortably again.

At that point, it would have been the easiest thing in the world to 'accept' that my time was up and fall into despair. Except, I am the kind of person who never gives up, whatever the circumstances. I find that this is the main difference between me and many others of my age (and younger!) – they give up too easily, are too fearful. They have decided – in their minds – that they are no longer as capable as they used to be.

I was determined not to let the doctors' prognosis bring my spirits down. I promised myself I would be out of the wheelchair as soon as it was humanly possible. In a little over two weeks, I was hobbling around the house using a walker. Ten days after that, about a month after I came home from the hospital, I was walking – a little unsteadily, perhaps, and slower than my usual brisk pace, but walking without aid. Today, of course, as you can see, I am fully and happily back to my old ways.

I had lost a lot of weight after my surgery. To stave off weakness and to put some weight back on, I began to eat breakfast after a lifetime of not doing so. Now I not only enjoy my daily breakfast but also, haha, lecture others on why they should not skip this most important meal.

The human body is so adaptable – it is the mind, with all its biases, fears and anxieties, that gets in the way. The body is also supremely intelligent – it knows what it needs at each stage of your life, and will not shy away from letting you know, if you only listen to it.

My advice to anyone of any age is: Don't ever say you *can't* do something – try believing that you have no idea what you are truly capable of, and see what happens!

'What does good health mean to me? To be able to do what I want to do. To be at peace with myself. To live joyfully.'

Like good physical health, good mental health can be cultivated. I have practised a few things in my life, some unconsciously, some deliberately, that have helped me stay content and be at peace.

One is never to compete or compare myself with others. I detest gossip like the plague – it usually comes down to putting someone down to make yourself feel better, which again can be traced to being competitive, in the unhealthiest way.

Another is not to obsess about or overthink anything. Ask yourself why everyone has to be analysed through *your* lens before you decide if they and their motivations are 'good enough', and you will find there is no good answer to that question. People are different – accept it and make your heart large enough to accommodate them. If their response to a situation is different from yours, try and see things from their point of view before deciding that you are right and they are wrong.

Trying to understand what makes people tick shapes my life. Letting them be who they are is my lifelong practice. It is very liberating – we unnecessarily burden ourselves with things when we can simply let go, understand, embrace. This acceptance that I have trained myself to feel has been the reason I have never rebelled against my circumstances or against people, whether as a child or a young woman, and that has kept me calm.

Stop living in fear. Ask yourself what is the worst thing that could happen and prepare yourself for it. You will come to realize that the worst outcome very rarely actually plays out. That realization, in itself, will help you become less fearful.

My father was a very generous person – he always appreciated people for good work. I have picked that up from him. You can only be genuinely appreciative of other people if you don't see yourself as being in competition with them. Generosity, whether you are dispensing material possessions, compliments or kindness, is such a great quality, because it fills both the giver and receiver with joy and love – I have tried all my life to cultivate it actively, and it has served me well.

I have often been told that I trust too easily, and that it is foolish and dangerous to do so. The children are kinder, they call it naïveté, and urge me to be more worldly-wise. But left to myself, I would always prefer to trust people until they do something to betray that trust. Even when they do, I do not dwell on it too long, or nurse a sense of injury – I have long ago realized that that kind of thing only harms me and my sense of well-being, not the perpetrator's.

People say that having a group of good friends, especially of your own age, is a big part of feeling happy and content. That is true for a lot of people, but not for me. I am not part of senior citizens' groups. I feel no need for companionship – I enjoy my own company. I feel blessed to be surrounded by my children and grandchildren; they are way younger than I am, and they keep me young.

For some years now, I have been part of a small, motley group of travel enthusiasts that go on short trips to lesser-known wildlife sanctuaries and places of natural beauty. I am, by far, the oldest in the group, but our similar interests and wavelength have helped us bond well with each other. These are not luxury trips, and we are all okay with that. All I really need when I travel is clean sheets, a clean, functional bathroom and good local food. We have travelled all over, and hiked in forests from Kashmir to Kerala – I feel very fortunate and privileged to be able to do things like this with people I like, by myself, even at 84.

Contentment can look like different things to different people, and can come from many different sources. I am at my most content when I can make other people happy, or even *see* other people being happy, even if I have nothing to do with it. I don't even have to know who they are – I may have spotted them from my window as they walk down the street, or they may be seated at the table across the room from me at a restaurant – but the sight of happy people brings me great joy.

Being amid nature is, as I have said before, another source of deep joy. I like growing things, whether on my balcony or in the small farm Milind has in Lonavala.

People may think that I have had it lucky, that they cannot feel the same sense of joy I do because their circumstances are very different. But **I truly believe that happiness is not something that happens to you; it is a choice that you make. Life is simple – it is we who complicate it.**

WHAT I TALK ABOUT WHEN I TALK ABOUT EATING

1. Eat slowly. It leads to good digestion and fills you with contentment.
2. Eat mindfully. Focus on what you are eating, savouring the different tastes and textures. Understanding that you are nurtured and nourished by what is on your plate brings reverence and gratitude.
3. Eat sitting down. Don't 'grab' food 'on the go'. It isn't respectful to the food, its growers and creators, or the physiological processes involved in eating.
4. Drink water after your meal. Warm water is great because it doesn't cause a shock to the system. Chilled water from the refrigerator is best avoided – I believe it makes you prone to cold and cough, especially if you drink it on a hot summer day.
5. Do not indulge in ritual fasting. It is better not to eat a lot in the first place.
6. Eat only when you are hungry. Many people today have no idea what it means to be hungry. They have never felt hunger because they are constantly eating – three proper meals, elevenses, something to munch on with chai, finger foods with a pre-dinner drink . . . it never stops.
7. Don't eat until you are full.
8. Don't eat something simply because you like it and therefore want it – think about whether you need it, at that point in time.
9. Don't eat once you've finished eating, simply because someone opened a packet of biscuits or a box of sweets or offered you a slice of fruit.

A DAY IN THE LIFE OF USHA

- I rise each morning around **5.45 a.m.**, and over the next hour, drink a litre of water while listening to the radio. After my surgery, I was advised to soak almonds and walnuts each night and eat them in the morning. I do want to do it, it's a good practice, but I usually forget to soak the nuts, and end up skipping them for the day.
- Around **7 a.m.**, having changed into a saree, I step out for my walk around Shivaji Park, and walk for a full hour.
- At **8 a.m.**, I make myself my first cup of chai, always adrakwali (ginger-laced) chai, with plenty of milk. I enjoy that cuppa with two or three biscuits. (I love biscuits – Marie biscuits, digestive biscuits, many other kinds of plain biscuits. Not cream biscuits, though – I find them too sweet.) I drink regular tea, I don't particularly like green.
- Around **9.30 a.m.**, we all have breakfast together. Breakfast is usually Indian – something simple like upma, poha or thalipith, which is a spiced Maharashtrian 'chapati' made with a mix of wheat, rice, bajra and jowar flours. You are meant to have thalipith with fresh-churned white butter, but we don't make butter at home, so we eat it with dahi instead.
- **Between 10.30 a.m. and 2 p.m.**, I read the morning newspapers end to end – this can take a while – and do a bit of cooking. There is someone to help me in the kitchen, but I prefer to do some of the cooking myself. I cook not with refined oil but with filtered oil. As long as my husband was around, I used sesame oil in the cooking, because he loved it; now I use peanut oil, which I love.

- We have lunch together around **2 p.m.** Rice is usually the carbohydrate, because Ankita much prefers it. Alongside, there will be some variety of dal (or usal with sprouts or pulses), two dry vegetables, of which one usually involves bhaji, or leafy greens, and a salad (koshimbir). Essentially, I cook and eat Marathi food, which I've eaten all my life. If Milind is eating lunch at home, he always wants khichdi, so that is also made for him.
- After lunch, I read or watch television. I doze off occasionally while watching TV, but it is always in my chair. I do not take afternoon naps – I find they ruin my digestion.
- My eldest, Netra, lives very close by. As part of her evening walk, she drops in for a cup of chai around **5 p.m**. I enjoy that second chai of the day while catching up with her very much. I do not have any biscuits or snacks with my evening cuppa. In fact, I don't snack between meals at all. I also do not drink aerated drinks, fruit juices, or anything out of a tetrapack.
- **Between 7 and 7.45 p.m.**, I attend an online exercise class that involves some yoga and stretches for mobility. It helps me very much.
- I eat my dinner around **8 p.m.** It's never a big meal, usually something like a bowl of soup or a glass of milk. If I'm not hungry, I simply skip it. The body's metabolism slows down with age, so it's better to eat less and not burden the system. At every meal, however, I am very particular about my posture – no slouching at the dining table! Sitting on the floor for eating is best, but I have never been able to sit cross-legged for some reason, so I sit at the table.
- Before the clock strikes **10**, I'm in bed for my 7.5 hours of shut-eye.

MILIND

From 'Keep Swimming' to 'Keep Moving'

'How we live our lives, for the most part, is based on our choices, not on our circumstances. Once you know what fulfils you, go out and do it.'

I ran my first half marathon, a distance of 21 kilometres, in 2004, at the age of 38. I had never run before, so in the months leading up to the run, I was happy to get advice from people who had been doing it awhile. It sounds incredible today, when we have the world's fastest growing running community in India, that even as recently as twenty years ago, running, as a lifestyle thing, was almost non-existent. Only serious athletes ran, or those in military training. It wasn't as if running was new to India, but we had only had professional runners before. Until the end of the nineteenth century, for instance, when the railways arrived and put them out of business, we had 'dak runners', who carried letters, messages and news from one town to another, armed with spears and knives to defend themselves against animals and bandits they encountered on the way. But that's a story for another day.

Back to the present. Part of the reason running has taken over India and the world today is economics and marketing – the American company Nike created a range of specialized 'running shoes' in the late '80s, and needed to sell them. It wasn't long before they set their sights on India. The company entered India through a licensing deal with an Indian partner in 1995; in 2004, Nike India set up shop. It was no coincidence that Procam announced the first Indian big-city marathon, open to anyone who cared to participate, in 2003.

Back then, everyone I asked advised me to train in a gym, on a treadmill. I did it for a few weeks, until I could run a decent distance continuously, during which time I realized how much I loathed being in a gym. Once the 10 kilometre mark had been breached, I quit the gym for the streets, never to return.

The big day dawned – it was the third Sunday of January. I had received dire warnings about all the things that could go horribly wrong while running the distance for the first time, and I was prepared for the worst. None of them came about – I ran the 21 kilometres comfortably, finishing in a little over two hours. I was ecstatic. Four months of good, healthy living, it seemed, had reversed years of abuse – my body had come through for me when I needed it to. Still, it would be another five years before I attempted the full marathon, at the age of 43. By then, I had improved my half marathon timing to an hour and 39 minutes, and was quite ready, I thought, for the full.

I could not have been farther from the truth. My progress in the 2009 Standard Chartered Mumbai Marathon, which was telecast live to the country because I was part of a reality show called *How To Run a Marathon*, turned out to be slow, painful and physically, mentally and emotionally gruelling. It was by far the toughest thing I had ever done.

But running my first marathon taught me, as every other experience so far had, a great deal about myself. More importantly, it validated some ideas that I had felt strongly about but had decided to put aside because the 'experts' thought differently. The prevailing expert wisdom on training for a debut marathon maintained that one should not attempt the entire marathon distance before the actual day, because that would tire the body out too much; there would not be enough time for recovery. 'Run 35 kilometres a couple of weeks before,' they said, 'and then taper off the distance until Marathon Day. On the day itself, the adrenaline rush of being cheered on by your home crowd and being surrounded by so many others attempting the same thing, will comfortably see you over the finish line.'

To me, that argument has always seemed illogical. Running 42 kilometres at a stretch is an insane feat of endurance for a human being – even dak runners passed their mail bags on to others every 15 to 20 kilometres and rested for the remainder of the day. If you haven't run the full distance before, ever, how can you be sure that you will be able to run it at all? Shouldn't you be running 50 kilometres in training, so that the 42 kilometres seem 'easy' in comparison? Will your mind not be far more at peace at the starting line then? After all, when one is engaged in such a demanding physical activity, when the body has reached the fag end of its reserves, isn't it your state of mind that makes the difference between success and failure? Still, out of respect to expert advice, I ran no more than 35 kilometres before the race.

My conviction that it was a bad idea was borne out by my experience during my first full marathon. As unexpected cramps paralysed my body, self-doubt about whether I would be able to last the course inundated my mind. I could have kicked myself for not having gone with my instinct.

From that day on, my innate scepticism for the wisdom of experts has only deepened. I listen to everything everyone says, cherry-pick what makes sense to me from their recommendations, even try them out for size, but in the end, I go with what I believe works for me.

I have benefited greatly from having been in competitive sport as a young man. Sport teaches you physical self-awareness. As a sportsperson, your focus is to never do anything that might cause you injury, because that could set you back by months. The moment you experience pain or discomfort, therefore, you try and resolve it, or simply stop doing what you are doing. That instinctive self-preservation response helps me when I put myself in uncomfortable situations of any kind – it ensures that I push myself in a 'comfortable way' and never go beyond what I know is good for me.

That knowledge, and my own self-belief, have allowed me to take on all manner of challenges in the last 15 years, all of which are well documented in press archives online and in my memoir *Made In India.* As always, it is not for records or glory or attention or to prove anything to myself that I do them, but simply to understand myself better, and hopefully, to inspire others to begin to believe in themselves, and to do the things they want to, comfortably. In 2012, at the age of 46, I ran the 1,500 kilometres from Mumbai to Delhi over 30 days, in the searing heat of May, to raise awareness about the environment as part of NDTV's Greenathon. At 50, I completed the Iron Man Triathlon, and followed it up with the Ultraman Challenge at 51.

In February 2014, I was in a nightclub in Chennai, as a favour to the hotel manager, who felt my presence would raise the club's cool quotient. That was when, shall we say, *I saw her standing there.* I was surprised at how intensely I felt drawn towards Ankita; that kind of thing does not happen to me often. It wasn't just that she was cute – I have spent my adult life surrounded by beautiful women, so I'm somewhat desensitized in that department. No, it was something else – a vibe, a certain attitude, that I found very attractive. Luckily, she came up to me to say hello. She was just 22, not 17, but seriously, *how could I dance with another*? Five years later, Ankita and I were married.

Two years after that, to celebrate my fifty-fifth birthday, I ran naked on a beach (and did not hesitate to post a long shot that Ankita took of the run, either!).

I do the things I want to and the things I'm comfortable doing, and I will do them as long as I am able. You may want to do other things, and you should go out and do them. When people ask what well-being means to me, I say it means being comfortable – in my body and in my head. Being comfortable in my body means being able to do any action – run, climb, squat, sleep, sit still – when I want or need to do it. Being comfortable in my head means being at peace, even in a difficult situation. There is nothing more important to me than this. Every decision I make and every action I take is geared towards achieving it.

No matter what it looks like to others, it isn't because I'm rich, or famous, or privileged, that I'm able to do the things I enjoy. I'm able to do them because I *choose* to do them. And so can you.

—

'The intelligence of any living being is constantly engaged in protecting and sustaining itself. If you don't care for your health, you are not intelligent. If you work against your own survival, you are not intelligent.'

Let's go back to experts for a bit. Sure, experts know a lot, but they know a lot about very little. The danger with going deep into a single area of specialization is that you lose sight of the big picture; you miss the wood for the trees. Specialists in the medical field run the greatest risk of that.

I'm often invited by doctors to talk to their professional groups about health and fitness. What I have discovered, to my alarm, is that while doctors know a lot about disease – how it looks, what is possibly causing it, how to treat it – they do not know much about health. I usually start my sessions by asking them a simple question – What is the biggest benefit of exercise? The answers I get, from people who understand intimately how the body works, are scarily similar to those of a layperson who skims the Sunday supplement of the daily newspaper. 'It helps you lose weight.' Or, 'It reduces stress levels.' Or, 'It releases endorphins that give you a happy high.'

I tell them what I think. 'Isn't the real benefit of exercise, of any kind of regulated movement, that it "wakes up" the different muscle groups in your body, that it improves your circulation? Isn't it right that good circulation is the only way to ensure that the nutrition and oxygen that we take in reaches every last cell of our bodies, so that they do not atrophy and die?' They nod thoughtfully, in assent. 'Now that you put it that way . . .' Such interactions have made me realize that while doctors are the people to go to when one is ill, one must look elsewhere for pointers on how not to fall ill, or how to support our immune system so that it is robust enough to hold off infection. And what better place to look, what more accessible laboratory for experimentation, empirical analysis and deduction than our own bodies?

The gathering of information, the following of cutting-edge research, the listening in to the opinions of experts in their fields – all this has now been made much, much easier via technology. If we are smart about navigating the web – in other words, if we search for information that can benefit us, instead of scrolling mindlessly and cluttering our minds with completely useless stuff, we can make better health decisions for ourselves. For instance, I have recently become interested in fasting as a way to rejuvenate the body. I looked for information on the internet and discovered a phenomenon called autophagy, a natural, evolutionary process of spring cleaning that the body does by removing damaged and dysfunctional parts of a cell. Autophagy works great when we are young, which is why most of us are naturally healthy when we are young, but as we get older, it slows down, causing dysfunctional cells to proliferate, causing disease. When cell debris isn't cleared regularly, it affects cell function, leading to ageing. One way to trigger autophagy as we get older, is fasting for over 18 hours at a time.

So far, all this is in the realm of experimental science – it hasn't been entirely accepted by the scientific and medical community. But there are enough studies that indicate that there could be something in this idea – enough to convince me to try it, anyway. I am a great believer in learning about myself by putting my body through controlled stress, so my attempt right now is fasting for 24 hours once a week to see if and how it affects me.

We bemoan the coming of social media, blaming it for allowing every vicious, agenda-driven, ignorant person in the world to air their opinion. In fact, we should be celebrating it. The wisdom of the crowd may well have helped humankind, with nary a fang or claw or talon to protect itself, survive as a species, and social media and rating apps are only the twentieth-century versions of it.

Social media has also brought back the great Indian tradition of questioning authority and challenging received wisdom. Personally, I want to hear what the 'trolls' have to say, for what they are doing is representing society and holding up a mirror to me in the process. People have always trolled me for not 'acting my age' or for marrying someone young enough to be my daughter. That doesn't make me feel hurt or angry, just curious. These people do not know me, their lives are not affected by me, and yet they feel justified in judging my choices and hating on me because it goes against their understanding of what is 'right' and 'good'. It makes me think of all the times I have been judgemental of others I don't know, in the same way. I now catch myself when I start being judgemental – it has helped me immensely to clear my own mind of negativity.

If we can stop getting 'triggered' by every person, every interaction, every experience, every situation that is not to our liking, and use each of them as ways to understand ourselves and the world better, we will live calmer, happier and therefore healthier lives

In the final analysis, isn't that the way we all want to live? And yet, we constantly, consciously, wilfully work against it. All too often, all too easily, we allow ourselves to lose sight of our long-term health goals for instant gratification. We tell ourselves that we are here to enjoy life, and that the way to do it is to indulge our palates – 'Biryani and daaru, boss, there's nothing more to life that that!' – and other appetites that are as seductive, as habit-forming, as detrimental to peace. Society supports and enables that kind of thinking, which makes it even harder to break away.

I would be the last person to refute the claim that we are put on this earth to enjoy life. We have been given the great gifts of our senses and emotions precisely so that we may enjoy it to the fullest, extracting the sweet, joyful rasa out of every moment. But to be able to do that, your mind must neither be churning with a million thoughts nor be made dull by intoxicants, pain or anxiety. The mind can be relaxed only if the body is relaxed, and the body is relaxed when it is working well, with all its systems chugging along as they are meant to. If you want to keep those systems in fine fettle, biryani and daaru, consumed unthinkingly and immoderately, are not the answer.

It is only a calm, undistracted mind that can focus with

laser-sharp clarity on the moment, and enjoy it to the fullest. This is also the biggest truth of sport. You can perform at your highest level only when you are at your most relaxed. When you swim competitively, you must focus all your energies, all your attention, not on winning, not on your opponent, not on the clock, but on getting the next stroke right. A perfect stroke is the greatest triumph. But it is over in a second, and now you have to focus on the next. That, to me, is meditation. That is the joy of the moment – to be in it fully, obsessively, as long as it lasts, and then to let it go, without regret, in the next.

This is what I believe at the end of 58 years of exploration. You do not have to believe it, or even agree with what I have said. You must go on your own journeys into charted or uncharted waters to understand yourself, and thereon, to discover what works for you.

It takes courage and cussedness to trust your own instinct, to believe that you are whole in and of yourself. But it is the only true way to live. When your thoughts are your own, and based on an understanding of yourself, there is no room for confusion or doubt. There is no one to blame and no one to owe allegiance to.

Try it for yourself. Walk the path that feels right to you, lonely as it may be, exploring each detour that comes along, seeing where it leads you. Follow the scent, follow your bliss and keep moving.

HOW TO EAT WELL, THE MILIND WAY

- **Always know where your food comes from.** If you aren't growing your own food, at least cook it yourself, so that you know what has gone into it. Can't cook? Get someone who loves you to cook you something. Not loved? Pay someone to cook for you, according to your instructions. Can't pay? Learn to cook!
- **Drinking water isn't the only way to hydrate.** All manner of fruits and vegetables also help – watermelon, cucumber, tomatoes and spinach, for example – as does coconut water. All these are also fortified by Mum Nature with essential vitamins and minerals.
- **If you have to eat processed food, pick foods processed using ancient techniques** like drying, salting, smoking or pickling in oil or brine. Tuck happily into dried fruit, seeds, nuts, salted meat, smoked cheese or gundruk, a side dish of fermented leafy veggies popular in Nepal and Sikkim. Avoid the mass-produced stuff, like biscuits.
- **Do not trust big corporations. Period.** All the stuff they say is good for you – protein drinks, vitamin supplements and more – are neither food nor medicine, and do not nourish or heal.
- **Balance – in food, movement and rest – is everything.** All food has potency, with the ability to harm or heal. The trick is in consuming what you do mindfully, and in moderation;

even water is harmful if you overdo it. The same applies to exercise and rest.

- **A little dirt goes a long way in making you strong.** When I was swimming competitively, one of our endurance tests was to swim from Sunk Rock, 5 kilometres out in the Arabian Sea, to the Gateway of India, through water thick with diesel, rotting vegetable matter, and actual sh*t. We did not come up smelling of roses, but it didn't make us sick. Some exposure to dirt and germs now and then, like an occasional plate of pani puri off a cart, will help your immune system stay in good nick.
- **Eat at least as sensibly as animals do.** We think of ourselves as a superior intelligence (here's an update: we're not) but while animals use their instincts to only pick food that is good for them, we abuse our bodies with foods we know are bad for us. Use your intelligence, not your emotions, when it comes to choosing your food.
- **Shitting well may be even more important than eating well.** Good digestion is the key to good health. If your body cannot digest the food you eat, if it cannot assimilate the nutrients contained in that food, the world's best diet will help you not a whit. Evaluate the benefits of what you eat not by the ease with which it enters your system but by the ease with which it leaves.

A DAY IN THE LIFE OF MILIND

- I wake up early, but lie in bed going through the messages and emails on my phone, before emerging around **9 a.m.**, after Aai and Ankita have returned from their morning walk and run. My breakfast, as anyone who follows me on social media knows, is a colossal amount of fruit. It takes care of all the hydration I need for the day.
- Until **11.30 a.m.**, or until the fruit is completely digested, I do other things – take care of bank work, make some calls. Around **11.30**, I may set out for a short run, after which I will head to Shivaji Park for 15–20 pull-ups on the bar. That should take no more than 5 to 7 minutes, but I could spend as much as 45 minutes in the Park, because that's where people find me and come up for a chat or to ask me for advice or a selfie.
- Before I sit down for lunch with the family around **2.30**, I do some push-ups, maybe a set of 40, just to know that I can still do it – if you don't use it, you lose it! It only takes me a couple of minutes. I only mention this so that readers see how easy it is to include a fitness routine (even if it lasts only two intense minutes) into your day. Lunch is usually Aai's ghee-fried khichdi (I have grown up on ghee and I love it), and an egg if I feel like it.
- **After lunch** is when I get to my real work. I might do my taxes and accounts, make my travel arrangements, schedule all the different things I do – speaking, film, photo and

ad shoots, interviews, modelling assignments, celebrity appearances at sporting events . . . I have no EA or secretary – I'm a bit of a control freak when it comes to my work, so I do it all myself. Most of my solo shoots are scheduled for the afternoon; if there are any happening that day, I head out to them. I get back home by 6 p.m. or a little later.

- Dinner is around **7.30 p.m.** Usually it is chapatis with two or three different kinds of vegetables, a salad and some dal. As an after-dinner treat, I sometimes have a chapati rolled up with ghee and jaggery – I adore it, and it satiates my massive sweet tooth. Of course, when I travel, and I travel for a big part of the year, I eat whatever is available. If I'm in India, however, I will definitely order khichdi at the hotel for at least one meal in the day.
- **Post-dinner**, I may catch a series or a movie on an OTT platform, before falling asleep around **11**. If I miss my 11 p.m. deadline, I will stay up until midnight, when a new Wordle puzzle drops on the *New York Times* app, and finish it before I sleep. I would like to sleep more, but I don't seem to need much sleep on a daily basis.

And that's my day – it's fairly ordinary, as you can see, involving no great physical feats, not even two hours in a gym, which many people imagine is a basic requirement for peak fitness. In fact, on most days, it is just the pull-ups and the push-ups, a total daily workout of 3 to 7 minutes max!

WHAT IS FITNESS? THE ABILITY TO ENJOY THE LIFE YOU HAVE MADE FOR YOURSELF

It is never too late to begin on your journey to fitness and good health. But there are some things to keep in mind when you do.

- **Before you begin, ask the important questions.** Ask yourself what good health means to you and why you want to be fit. Whatever your answers, fashion a life and lifestyle that aligns with them. Do not compare your exercise routine to anyone else's – their motivations for working out (getting a six-pack) may be very different from yours (trekking to 14,000 feet comfortably).
- **Start slow and gradual, but start regular.** If you've never been sporty, and have just decided to jump on the fitness bandwagon, be very mindful of your pace. If you're panting during a run, you're running too fast. If you're exhausted after a run, you've run too much. Try different things, at your level, to gain an understanding of your body's capabilities before you ramp it up. But whatever you pick, do it every single day.
- **Mix it up a bit.** From time to time, push yourself out of your comfort zone and try something new. If you are a good runner, add yoga a couple of times a week. If swimming is what you like, go cycling every Sunday. In your side fitness hustle, focus on the movement you don't get as part of your main exercise routine.

- **You don't have to do a hundred different kicks each day.** While it is good to mix things up, doing the same 'kick' (read: routine) over and over, like Jaden Smith in *The Karate Kid*, brings mastery, calm and a deeper understanding of your body.
- **Pick one thing you cannot do and pursue it sincerely – rest assured, the results will come.** Exercise is not about punishing the body. It is about being comfortable in it while coaxing it, day after day, to explore what it can do. I have been trying to do a split for a year now. After months of pushing my body a teeny bit further each day, I am, finally, almost there.
- **Work regularly on the movements against gravity – pulling, hanging, jumping, leaping, balancing, which children are able to do so easily.** These are the ones you lose the ability to do, as you age, if you do not practicse them. Pushing and squatting are easier – we lose those movements last.
- **Review your fitness routine periodically** to see if it is working for you – are you closer to your fitness goals six months into the routine than you were before you began? What has the routine taught you about yourself? Do you need to change or tweak the routine because of what you have learnt?
- **Pay attention to your body's speed of recovery. It is a better measure of your fitness than how much weight you can lift.** So is its ability to adapt to new and unexpected situations and circumstances.

- **Even if you are not training for an event, make sure you keep moving.** There is a difference between training and conditioning. Conditioning is ensuring that you put aside some time each day, even ten minutes, for some kind of movement – pull-ups, push-ups, a short run or brisk walk, some suryanamaskars. Training is when you ramp up the exercise with a particular event in focus – a race, a hike, or some other physical challenge. If your body is not conditioned, you are more likely to suffer an injury when you begin training.
- **Don't worry too much about speed.** Personally, I want to be able to run 100 kilometres over two days, all my life – why should I run at any particular speed? The Japanese slow running technique called Niko Niko – Smile Smile, is about jogging at a 'smiling pace', slower than you walk, and it is more difficult than you would expect. As a rule of thumb, finishing comfortably – can you have a conversation with someone right after you cross the finish line? – is finishing strong.
- **Focus on your weaknesses.** If you have weak joints, do exercises that strengthen the muscles and tendons and ligaments around them. Neglect to do this, and the weaker parts will keep deteriorating while the stronger ones compensate for them, until they too break down. Your strengths should prop up your weaknesses, your weaknesses should not pull down your strengths.

- **Don't over-rely on tech.** Wearable monitors, activity trackers and other devices give you the illusion of being on top of things, but they make you so dependent on them that you begin to second-guess your own instinct when it comes to your health. There is nothing more dangerous. Use them if you must, but rely more on your body's signals.
- **When in doubt (and even when not) do suryanamaskars.** If you aren't quite sure what fitness routine is for you, spend five to ten minutes a day doing a few suryanamaskars, at a slow pace, focusing on form and breathing in each posture. By the time you become comfortable in every posture, and can hold each for five breaths, you will be fit.

ANKITA

Finding Equilibrium in the Ebb and Flow

'It is never too late to begin cultivating a good relationship with your body. But do it respectfully, honouring your own body's needs. The idea of "whipping" your body into shape, whether you are 20 or 50, is inherently violent and disrespectful.'

Once I began to eat better and feel better in my head, I was inspired to move a little more, and more regularly. I bought myself my first smart watch, with the aim of clocking 10k steps a day. Then I bought another smart watch, so that I could listen to uninterrupted music off the second watch while the first tracked my route using the GPS, without either of them running out of juice. I even joined a gym. With my hardware in place, I was all set to turn into a fitness diva. It was not January, but I was full of the first-week-of-the-year enthusiasm that marks a grand new resolution.

Needless to say, like most new year resolutions, this one soon floundered. I did hit the gym when I could and I did take walks around the boundary of my housing society in Dwarka, New Delhi, where I lived then, but I was not able to be as regular as I had hoped. The airline schedules were crazy, which messed up my circadian rhythms and sleep patterns, but the real problem was one of motivation. I did not particularly enjoy going to the gym; it was something I felt I needed to do to be fit, but not much else. As for walking, I soon realized it wasn't half as much fun when I was doing it to a plan, to complete a number-of-steps target, as it had been when I was in college, when I walked simply because I had all the time in the world and wanted to be with my music and my thoughts. Plus, walking in a giant, densely populated, polluted metropolis is a very different experience from walking in a small, hilly town.

I might have gone on like this indefinitely, even while dating one of the country's biggest fitness icons, if not for another phone call. This one was from my sister, Maina, somewhere around October 2016. She had called to tell me that she was pregnant.

A shock of excitement ran through me. I was going to

be an aunt! This was big news, and I had to figure out how to deal with it. I was elated, but also vibrating with nervous energy, like I do when I have a cup of coffee (sadly, even though I love coffee, I have it very seldom, because it makes me jumpy). Not sure what to do but knowing that I had to work that energy out of my system before I could begin to think clearly, I headed for the gym. But that day, for some reason, the gym was shut.

I considered, and decided it did not matter. I was already in my workout attire – I might as well 'work out' on the street if not in the gym. Jittery as heck, I began to run, my music turned off, my head exploding with thoughts. A brand-new little person, who knew nothing about me, was coming into my life. He or she would be watching me, learning from me, *judging* me. I would be part of that little person's closest family, one of the biggest early 'influencers' in his life – if I hoped for him or her to think well of me, I had to damn well make sure I was a great one. It was a huge responsibility. In other words, it was time to clean up my act.

When I stopped running 6 kilometres later – as recorded by my smart watch, in case you were wondering – I felt no exhaustion, just happiness. It had as much to do with the news of my nephew's impending arrival as with the run itself. In the course of those 40 minutes, I had recaptured for myself something that had been missing from my life lately – the sheer joy of locomotion, the freeness of mind and the feeling of liberation that comes from feeling your body do what it does best – move.

There was nothing to stop me now from keeping my daily date with movement – I was on! Suddenly, I was finding the time to run. I ran before I left for work, or after I came back, or in the middle of the workday when I caught a break. I ran at dawn, mid-morning, noon or evening, whenever a slot presented itself. The very next month, in November 2016, I ran my first 10k at the Mumbai Pinkathon and completed it in an excellent debut time of 64 minutes. Just three months later, I took part in a half marathon, and placed third! It was ridiculous – I had never run long distance in my life, and here I was, covering 21 kilometres without breaking a sweat (metaphorically speaking), and loping to a podium finish, with almost no 'training'! It seemed that my legs, which had walked and pedalled me over so many thousands of kilometres over the years, had fallen back easily, joyfully, into the familiar, well-practised rhythms of my childhood and youth, and were showing me the many ways in which they could help me heal, and find joy, power, strength, courage and self-belief on the way there. I could not have been more grateful.

'Many fitness goals are so short-sighted and so visual – six-pack abs, for instance, or a flat stomach. The real goal of exercise is to make you happy, confident, content – a better version of yourself.'

In 2018, Milind and I were married. It had been a bit of a battle convincing my parents to accept him as a potential son-in-law, but they had come around in the end. They knew, as I did, that I would never go against their wishes, but they also knew that I would not marry anyone else. Mamma was concerned about the vast difference in our ages; Papa worried that, being an actor, he would have starry airs and would not fit in with the family. But when Milind first visited my parents in Guwahati, Papa discovered that he was quite happy wearing the same pair of jeans for a whole week and tramping about in the same Lunas whether we were going on a hike or to a formal event. He was not fussy about food either and did not need anything fancy – his go-to meal was, and continues to be, a simple khichdi. I knew Papa's approval was complete when he began teaching himself Marathi. I was over the moon – if there was one person in the world I never wanted to hurt, it was Papa.

I quit my job a couple of months before the wedding. Our hectic travel schedules had seen to it that Milind and I had spent very little time together in the four years that we had been a couple; I saw no point in having that state of affairs continue even after we were married. Plus, I really, really wanted to hit the pause button on being 'responsible' for a while, sink back into days that had no timetables and targets, and think, with no pressure, about what I wanted to do with my life.

The first year of our marriage was a dazzling whirl of travel, running, hiking, and . . . my very first full marathon! What made it even more goosebump-worthy than it might have been was that it happened in . . . Athens! Yes, on 12 November 2018, a little over two years since I had first started running, Milind and I ran the Athens Classic Marathon (The Authentic), which ends at the historic Panathenaic Stadium, where a racetrack was first built in 330 BC to host the Panathenaic Games, the precursor to the modern Olympics! The best part? It wasn't even planned!

That November, Milind and I were in Greece on a holiday, to celebrate his birthday. Now, this kind of thing – a getaway to celebrate a special occasion – may seem commonplace for most couples in their first year of marriage, but it was a very unusual thing for us. You see, my husband did not understand the concept of travelling for leisure; he had never done it. He only travelled for work – a shoot, a running or fitness event, a motivational talk that he had been invited to deliver. There was so much of that happening that his idea of a holiday, of spending some precious couple time together, was to stay at home in Mumbai. That didn't matter a whit to me – I was having a year-long honeymoon, visiting all kinds of wonderful places that I had never seen before, and I was delighted.

But I still wanted to make his first birthday as a married man special, and that's how the Greece trip came up. It was only after we had got there that we discovered that the Athens Classic Marathon was happening soon. Needless to say, Milind wanted to run it. I could not deny the birthday boy such a treat in his birthday week, so I acquiesced. He proposed I run it too, along with him, since it was more about the thrill of running the 'original' marathon, not about whether I would be able to finish. As it turned out, I did cross the finish line! It was the biggest thrill of my life.

That year was also about taking on other brand-new challenges, like scuba diving. That may not seem like something to make such a fuss about, but if you were me – my husband had been the national swimming champion and national record-holder in his category for many years as a young man and had completed both the Ironman and the Ultraman Triathlons in his 50s, while I, um, did not know how to swim – you would see why this was a triumph of mind over matter.

In this way, month after month, plugged into Milind's insane travel schedule, we went from city to city, and continent to continent, relentlessly. And it was all hunky-dory. At least in the beginning.

As the months rolled by, however, despite my best efforts to stay excited, it all began to get a little overwhelming for me. I wanted to hit the pause button all over again.

I was bewildered. This was, technically, the happiest time of my life. I was married to someone who loved me deeply and who I adored. My family loved him, his family loved me. I was living my dream of travelling to exotic destinations for leisure. I was finally beginning to get over the trauma of K's death, and I had an adorable new nephew. I was eating well, moving well, being good, feeling good. And yet, and yet, some anxiety had begun to resurface. I felt unmoored, not in control. After a particularly hectic period of haring from one city to another for weeks on end, I felt I simply could not take it anymore. Feeling completely disloyal, I told Milind I would like to stay on in the last hotel for a few more days, all by myself, while he returned home to Mumbai. He shrugged. 'Sure, do whatever you feel like.'

For three days, I vegetated in the hotel room, lying on the bed, meeting no one, ordering room service for every meal, staring at the ceiling for hours, my mind a blank. I did not run, I did not stretch, I hardly moved. It was wonderful. I realized, once again – if this is beginning to sound repetitive, trust me that this is how the process goes; iteration after iteration in the same loop, getting a wee bit closer to the truth each time – that even in the midst of such happiness with my partner and our families, what I truly craved, and missed, was time with myself. That was when the other epiphany happened, the one I hadn't allowed myself to acknowledge – all the running I was doing was tiring me out. My body felt wrung out, stiff, at the end of a long run, not full of life and vitality. I needed to fix it.

That was how I came to yoga. That was how, however cheesy this sounds, I found myself again.

People think that yoga is about postures, but what it has taught me is how to breathe. I know what you're wondering – why does anyone need to be 'taught' how to breathe? – but it is the truth. Yoga postures are important because they 'awaken' the body, and get the prana, or vital energy, flowing. 'Holding' postures trains the body not to fidget. But that stillness in body, which eventually leads to stillness of mind, cannot be achieved without breathing right.

Learning to breathe right has helped me immensely with my running – earlier, I thought nothing of breathing through my mouth when I ran, and that used to tire me out. Now I only breathe through my nose, the way yoga taught me to. If you think about it, there is something unnatural about breathing through the mouth – if we were meant to do that, there would be 'filters' in our throats as well, as we have in our noses. The advantage of nose breathing is not only that it conserves energy, but it also works as a barometer – as long as I am able to breathe comfortably through my nose while I'm running, I know I'm doing okay.

When you are pushing your body, you can only go beyond a certain limit if you are acutely aware of your breathing and are able to moderate it. The awareness of the breath that I learnt through yoga has helped me do things like learning to scuba dive without fear, when I did not even know to swim. It is also responsible, I firmly believe, for helping me complete a 1 kilometre distance in the water just two months after I first began to learn. More than anything else, yoga brought me the calmness I sorely needed.

It was exactly the kind of support and direction I required at the time. I went back to my running, and everything else I had been doing, with new energy, and a new understanding of why I was doing it – it wasn't to impress my husband, it wasn't for my ego, it wasn't because I wanted six-pack abs. I was running simply because I loved it, and because I owed it to my beautiful body.

'Milind is a huge influence on me where health and fitness are concerned, but all my insights are my own, through the lived experience of my body. You are the only person who can decide what is good for you.'

Once I began to run 'well' – breathing naturally during the run and healing well after, both gifts of my yoga practice – it seemed I could not stop. I stopped plugging into my music while I ran and let my mind wander instead. At best, I listened to calming chants before the race, which helped to centre me. My yardstick for how good my run had been was no longer my finishing time – I stopped chasing things like that – but whether my breathing had been good enough for me to be able to talk to someone comfortably right after I ran past the finish line.

In 2018, I ran alongside Milind in The Last Long Run – an annual tradition he had created for himself where he ran from place X to place Y on the last two days of the year, before bringing in the new year at place Y. That year, we ran the 140 kilometre distance between Colombo and Unawatuna in Sri Lanka; only two weeks later, I ran the Tata Mumbai Marathon, very comfortably. In 2019, I became possibly the first Assamese woman (I put this out on my social media then, and no one has challenged me yet) to summit Kilimanjaro.

Full of energy, I also began training at a shooting range – and found I was naturally good at the sport. In any case, it was a great way to channel any residual negative energy – I realized, for the first time, how cool I felt, how invincible, with a gun in my hand. That set off the alarm bells in my head. I slowly weaned myself off the shooting – depending on something external to feel powerful is a bad idea; the trick is to find the invincible on the inside.

Towards the end of 2017, Papa retired, and my parents came back to their Guwahati home. Just two years later, my father's kidneys began to fail, from Type 2 diabetes, which he had lived with for several years. The doctor who first saw him was shocked at his glucose levels, which were well above 500. My dad, like Milind's, did not believe in doctors and allopathic medicine. Throughout our childhood, Maina and I were taken only to the homoeopath when we were ill, unless we had to get our eyes or teeth checked. My dad had always dealt with his diabetes by drinking bitter gourd juice and chewing on methi seeds, believing that they would see him through.

They didn't. In early 2020, Papa's kidneys failed completely, making him dependent on dialysis three times a week simply to stay alive. Personally, I think it was all the stress he had taken on over the decades – trying to be honest within a corrupt system, ensuring that his daughters got a good education while worrying about them being on their own, making sure that Mamma was always comfortable – manifesting itself in this way in his body. I think his body held on not only until both his daughters were married, but until he was convinced that they were happy in their marriages. Then, heaving a sigh of relief, it let go.

When the dialysis phase began, Papa lost all will to live. For reasons he never explained to us, he was very sure he did not want anyone else's organs inside his body. Without a new, improved life to look forward to, he began to fade fast. Mamma, who had devoted herself to his care since the first damning diagnosis, continued to wear herself out looking after him, which may also have added to his stress. The end came in early 2021, in the ICU of the hospital that had been looking after him. I was on hospital duty that night and in the elevator trying to get to the ICU when my beloved Papa left us. It was close to midnight, and I didn't see the point of rousing Maina or Mamma at that time. Instead, I closed his eyes, placed cotton wool in his ears and nostrils, and volunteered to accompany his body to the morgue in the basement.

There was no one else in the elevator. My mind was a whirl, listing out all the tasks that I had to immediately get on to after depositing him in the morgue, wondering how I would break the news to my family, wanting to get all of this done quickly and systematically. When we were between floors, the elevator stopped, for no apparent reason. All my fretting did not make it start moving again. I gave up. This was entirely out of my control, and there was nothing I could do. I looked at Papa's peaceful face properly for the first time since his death, my mind suddenly empty. As if on cue, all the gratitude I felt for having had him in my life came pouring out. I told him how proud I was to be his daughter, I told him what a great dad he had been. Only when I had done this did the elevator begin to move again. My Papa had made sure I said a proper goodbye to him, because he knew that I would always regret it if I didn't. It was surreal.

Mamma went to pieces. She was still young, only 54, but her married life, and particularly the last few years of it, had revolved entirely around Papa. This time, it was me, her youngest, who, having once let her own life slide so spectacularly in the aftermath of another loss, took on the role of coach and mentor to pull Mamma out of her misery. I cannot deny that it helped enormously to have, within the family itself, a towering figure to serve as inspiration.

'Look at Aai!' I often scolded Mamma in the months that followed, while Maina begged me to be less aggressive. 'She is 80, and she doesn't think of herself as old, ever. And look at you, behaving like your life is over. Papa was only part of your life, Mamma, there is so much more of you for you to discover. Get out, do things, take up a hobby, start doing something for yourself.'

By and by, she emerged from her grief. Today, she has taken up yoga and enjoys going on little hikes and treks with her grandchildren, who, like all children, are also brilliant role models for how to live curiously, joyously, in the moment.

As for me, I am a work in progress, as are we all. I continue walking the path towards healing and empowerment, and am on a mission to bring other women into the fold. Towards the end of 2022, I came up with the idea of Invincible Women's Run, a women-only event that offers both the long-distance format – 50, 75 and 100 kilometres – and the short distance format – 3, 5 and 10 kilometres – to participants to choose from. On 18 and 19 February 2023, Milind flagged off its inaugural edition, which had over 2,500 women take part, in Mumbai. I hope to keep this going, adding fun runs like the Saree Run, the Grandmothers' 10k, the Baby-wearing Moms' Walk, and more into the mix, apart from inspirational runs, like one featuring only cancer survivors.

Having experienced for myself, in glorious large-format Kodachrome, the positive impact of physical activity on mental health, it would be selfish not to invite other women to experience it too.

If I am talking about making a difference, can yoga be far behind? On International Yoga Day 2023, I launched Atmabodha by Ankita (atmabodhabyanki.com), an initiative to get more and more people to experience the beauty, power and joy of yoga. I had been meaning to do something in this direction ever since I got my yoga teacher certification in 2021, and I'm thrilled that it has finally happened.

Who knows what the future holds? I have experienced how life can change in a minute, from dazzling bright to utter dark, and how, if you persist and persevere, it will change back to dazzling, even if the texture of the light is different. The only truth is that the power to change it from one to the other lies not outside of you, but inside. Always.

MY MANTRAS FOR HOLISTIC HEALTH

- **Learn to listen to the voice inside you** – But which voice? Beware of the big voice that insists you cannot do something. Focus on the smaller voice saying, 'Mayyyyyyybe you can? How can you be sure until you try?'
- **Allow yourself to feel things wholly, completely.** If you need to have a loud, ugly cry in the middle of the day, do it. If you are feeling happy, dance even if you are a bad dancer. Let your body help you express your mind.
- **Make time to be with nature.** Walk barefoot – on the grass, in the mud, in water. Connect with the earth.
- **Move, move, move.** You have heard it before, but there is nothing truer – regular physical activity leads to better mental health. Better mental health helps you take better care of your body.
- **Respect your fears, as long as they are useful.** Instead of letting your fears paralyse you, examine them to see how you can make them useful. For instance, fear of a worst-case situation can help you prepare better for it. If you cannot make use of a fear, let it go.
- **You become your thoughts.** Your thoughts are fashioned out of what you consume – physically, mentally, emotionally. Be very mindful of what kind of stimulation, and how much of it, you provide your mind.

- **The questions 'Why do we eat?' and 'Why do we exercise?' have only one right answer each:** I eat because I want to get healthier, I exercise because I want to get stronger. Burn these into your brain.
- **Practise yoga – it is a regimen that exercises every muscle from fingertip to toe-tip.** Plus, the breathing techniques involved in yoga not only ensure that your body gets enough oxygen but also that your mind becomes calm, less impulsive, less emotional.
- **Add Vedic chants to your yoga practice.** The vibrations the chants set off inside you will help you centre yourself and reboot, bringing your body and mind back into alignment.

MY THOUGHTS ON FOOD, EATING AND HEALING YOUR BODY

- **Any food that makes your body happy and comfortable, throughout the digestive process, is a superfood.** Energy bars list many ingredients that are considered superfoods, but most such bars taste like cardboard. For a quick burst of energy, eat familiar foods like dates, raisins, jaggery, a bit of chocolate, chikki, oranges, bananas and roasted peanuts instead.
- **Eat the foods that your body craves, but in moderation – they indicate what your body needs.** Some of us are drawn naturally to sweet foods, others to spicy or salty foods. We tend to overeat such foods because of our hunter-gatherer genetic programming, which urges the body to stock up whenever those foods become available. Break that programming not by denying your body what it craves but by feeding it just enough of it to make it feel secure.
- **Make the faculty of smell your ally.** My grandfather used to say 'ghranam ardha bhojanam', which is Sanskrit for 'Half (the satisfaction) of eating lies in the smelling'. I love coffee, but it doesn't suit me, so I trick my mind into getting its coffee high from smelling it brewing. I eat Maggi noodles once a year as a special treat, but get my Maggi high from every roadside kiosk I pass that is cooking it. Win-win!

- **Alcohol is bad for you. Period.** I've been there and done that and there is *no* debate about it. I truly do not understand 'beer runs' and other such strange practices. After a long run, your body is already very vulnerable. Instead of pampering it with water and fortifying, nourishing food, why would you abuse it with beer?
- **Drink water when you are thirsty.** How much water should you drink in a day? As much as *you* need! Some of us are dinosaurs and some are butterflies – how can the 'three litres a day' rule work for both?
- **Review your food practices regularly.** At the moment, I comfortably run 10k without drinking water before or during because my body doesn't seem to need it. That may change, will change, as my body changes. It is silly to stick to rituals that worked for you at 30 when you turn 40 or even 34, without checking from time to time that they are still working.
- **Trust the body's natural ability to heal itself.** Rest, sleep, nourishing food, natural remedies – those are usually all the body needs to support it through mild illnesses. I grew up chewing on tender parijat leaves to bring down a fever, tender guava leaves and pickled lemon to soothe stomach cramps and bananas to cure mild diarrhoea.

A DAY IN THE LIFE OF ANKITA

Okay, before we get into this, a disclaimer – there is no typical day in my life. Maybe it is my age, but I abhor routine. I find it tiresome to have a regulated timetable or activity schedule for the day, and I like to take life as it comes.

- I wake up most mornings around **5.30**. Sitting in silence, I tap my body from head to toe, appreciating each part as I go. The tapping stimulates the different muscle systems and pressure points and 'wakes them up'.
- Before I get out of bed, I finish any water remaining in the 1.5 litre bottle by my bedside, which I fill up before I go to sleep.
- Once I have freshened up, I do some yoga stretches to get all the kinks out of my spine and shrug off whatever stress I have stored in my neck, back and hips the previous day. After that, if I'm feeling calm and collected, I will continue with a full yoga routine followed by some meditation. If I'm a little anxious or jumpy, I go for a run instead. For me, running works like a different kind of meditation. Then more yoga stretches and some pranayama.
- By **9 or 9.30 a.m.**, I'm ready for the first meal of the day – usually fruit and an egg and toast. I may also add some almonds and walnuts or some moong that I have soaked the previous night and a bit of whatever Aai has made for breakfast.

- About an hour after eating, if I feel like it, I may go for a swim. If not, I will shower, get dressed – I have no beauty routine, and I don't use make-up, so this takes two ticks – and get on with my day. If I have work to do or a yoga class to teach, I get to it. If I'm feeling gloomy or anxious, I sit down to write – a song, a poem (that is not necessarily poetic, haha), my feelings – it helps me clarify my thoughts. I may read, solve a crossword puzzle, play my guitar (I've just picked up a ukelele I'm trying to master), help Aai with something. If I'm missing home, I will order fish or chicken and cook it for myself the Assamese way.
- I like to sleep early, so my social outings are always around lunchtime. At restaurants, I usually eat something simple, not very spicy or heavy. All my years in hostel have made me unfussy about food – I like different tastes and am happy to experiment. If I'm eating meat, I order a salad on the side – I like to know that I'm getting enough fibre into my diet.
- I don't nap in the afternoon, so I'm usually out running errands or checking out a new store or something. In the evening, if I'm around, I will have a cup of tea with Aai. I eat dinner around **7 p.m.**, but only if I am hungry, and do not eat after **8 p.m**. if I can help it.
- **10 p.m**. is lights out. It works for me and for everyone else around me as well – I am not nice to people if I haven't slept enough!

THE SOMAN SUTRA: WE EAT WHAT MAKES OUR BODIES SING – THEY'RE NOT ALWAYS THE SAME THINGS

FRUIT

Usha: Milind insists that fruit should only be had in the morning on an empty stomach, but I don't go very much by that. Logically, your stomach becomes empty three hours after a meal, so if you eat fruit then, you ARE eating on an empty stomach! Unlike Milind, I'm not a big fan of fruit – I eat a small banana or two sometimes, or a bit of jackfruit, mango, sitaphal or chikoo in season.

Ankita: My husband and fruit! Anyone who follows him on Instagram knows how much of it he eats. As for me, I can't eat too much fruit – it sets up an uncomfortable tingling in my body. So I'm usually just picking at something to give him company.

Milind: What can I say? I love fruit! One whole watermelon and one whole papaya at breakfast are de rigueur, to which I will add whatever fruit is in season – 5–6 mangoes, a couple of avocados, 2–3 dragon fruit . . .

MEAT

Usha: I don't eat meat any more, don't even cook it at home – I find it difficult to digest now. I love fish, though, so I do eat it occasionally, and sometimes prawns as well.

Milind: I've been trying to give up meat because I personally believe it isn't healthy, but I haven't succeeded so far. I grew up eating mutton, but my favourite meat is pork. Not the biggest fan of cold cuts, sausages or bacon, though.

Ankita: I love pork and silkworm, but I only have those when I'm home in Guwahati. I don't buy or cook pork in Mumbai because I feel it doesn't have the same quality as back home.

WATER

Usha: I have a whole litre soon after I wake up in the morning. That's my only water ritual. For the rest of the day, I drink when I am thirsty.

Milind: Only about half a litre of water a day, and that is because Ankita insists I must. (As for alcohol, she allows me three beers and two shots of Sambuca a year.)

Ankita: Oh, I drink a LOT of water through the day – it's very important to me. I drink water through the night as well.

THE SWEET STUFF

Usha: I love Indian sweets! I don't think I would ever give them up, but I use discretion in how much and how often I eat them.

Milind: I love, love, love sweets, especially jalebi. To cut down on processed sugar, I try to eat sweets made of jaggery whenever possible. I adore chocolate, but I eat much, much less of it than

I used to. I fool my sweet tooth into thinking I've had dessert by eating things like hung curd with honey or goat cheese with honey.

Ankita: In general, I don't like sweet things very much. In fact, I'm partial to bitter things – karela, neem leaves sautéed in a little oil and seasoning for an evening snack, moringa leaves bhaji with aloo . . .

THE SOMAN SUTRA: HOW TO REDUCE DRAMA IN YOUR LIFE

Usha: Be patient. It is the single most important ingredient to staying calm. Be patient with situations – don't react to provocation, don't expect quick solutions. Be patient with people – you have no idea what they are going through. Be patient with yourself when you're trying to cultivate a new habit, like starting a fitness regimen. Patience also helps you sit with a situation, analyse it and learn from it. That introspective pause will help reduce your regret, grief, anger. In other words, less drama.

Milind: Know what you want with crystal clarity – it will help you cut out from your life things that you do not want, i.e., things that cause drama. I know that I do not want to deal with conflict, so I avoid it like the plague. If I sense that a new project or business will at some point lead to conflict, I turn it down, no matter how much fame, money or social cachet is involved. That gives me the mindspace to pour my energies into the things that I care about, like family and my own well-being. It is as simple as that. Most people struggle with decision-making and then go on to regret the decisions they made because they are confused about what they want in the first place.

Ankita: Communicate! If you don't like something someone said or did to you, or if you are hurt by it, let them know, politely but firmly. Don't expect them to realize it by themselves – they may have done it unknowingly, or, in their worldview, their action may not be problematic. If you have a bad reaction to it and bottle it up, it will come out, at some point, in a toxic way, and it will lead to drama. There will usually be a solution if you communicate, but if there isn't, you can tell yourself you tried, get closure and move on.

EPILOGUE

When three remarkably thoughtful and articulate people have had their say, there is nothing much left to add. Except, perhaps, to go back to the very beginning of the book, to the questions in the first paragraph, and check if, having now been part of three inspiring journeys, we are surer of the answers. Maybe it is helpful to read through the rest of that introductory chapter, and now that we know their stories, reflect on how each of the three exemplify the well-being 'non-rules' listed there, in very specific and unique ways, in their own lives. And maybe now it's time to stop reading and start doing.

'Hey,' says Milind, 'I have a great idea for the closing chapter. Have you heard of the Proust Questionnaire? No? Well, in nineteenth-century Europe, among the elite, a sort of parlour game used to be played when the family had guests to dinner. A so-called 'confession album' would be produced, and the guest would be asked to fill in a set of questions in it. Questions like – your favourite qualities in a man/woman, your chief characteristic, your favourite virtue, your main fault, your idea of happiness, your idea of misery and so on. The answers, some of which required some soul searching, were supposed to reveal the guest's 'true personality'.

'In 1924, two years after the death of the celebrated French writer Marcel Proust, a confession album in which Proust had answered a set of questions was discovered. A French literary journal published Proust's page from the album as its lead story, and it went absolutely viral. The idea of a questionnaire that revealed one's most secret thoughts was picked up by journalists for their celebrity interviews, and later by schoolchildren, who passed around confession albums for their friends to fill up. Because it was so closely associated with Marcel Proust, the questionnaire began to be called the Proust Questionnaire, even though he had nothing to do with framing the questions.'

Good for Proust! What does this have to do with the Big Idea for this book's closing chapter?

'Well, what if I came up with a version of the Proust Questionnaire for the readers of this book? They can take as much time as they need to answer it, but the very individual, very specific answers the questions will elicit will help readers understand themselves and their fitness and health motivations better. That clarity will ensure that they not only begin but also sustain their fitness journeys. As I have said so many times in the book, a fitness journey is really a self-awareness journey, and this questionnaire will help readers kick-start the latter. Sounds like a plan?'

It certainly does! Let's go!

The Soman 'Your True Fitness Personality' Questionnaire

1. What do I want in life, I mean, really-really? What am I willing to compromise on – health, wealth, family, sleep – to get it?
2. What do I consider the FIVE most important things in life *(rank by order of priority from 1 to 5)*?
3. Is good health on my list of Five Most Important Things? If not, why? If yes, proceed to the next question.
4. Why do I want to be healthy? *(Write your reasons down. As many as you can think of. Then put them all down on a large poster and hang it up on your wall, where you can see it. Every day.)*
5. What am I prepared to commit to, to ensure my health and well-being?
6. Why do I eat? What does food mean to me? Why do I (not) exercise? What does exercise mean to me?
7. What are my GOOD food and fitness habits? What are

my NOT-SO-GOOD food and fitness habits? Which do I practise more?

8. What are my biggest challenges to maintaining good physical and emotional health? *(The challenges could be personal, circumstantial, professional, social. Once you have listed them down, ask yourself the same question again and strike out items from your list that are really excuses. Rinse and repeat.)*
9. What is one challenge I am grappling with right now that is preventing me from moving forward? Is there some way to move past it? If yes, why haven't I done it so far? If no, why am I still treating it as a challenge instead of accepting it as my reality and moving on?
10. How long has it been since I tried something that is entirely out of my comfort zone? *(If your answer is 'too long', maybe it's time to do something to change that.)*

'This is by no means an exhaustive list of questions,' clarifies Milind. 'These are just prompts to get you going. The rest of the questions – and they will be different for different people – will emerge as you answer these. Here's a tip – Be brutally honest when you answer. Own the answers without judgement. It isn't *what* your answers are that matters, it is the fact that you have reflected seriously on the questions. Right, are you ready? Well then, get set and go!'

There's the starting gun, folks! The book is done, but the journey is just beginning. Start strong, stay centred and keep moving.

 @keepmoving 

  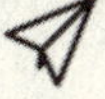 

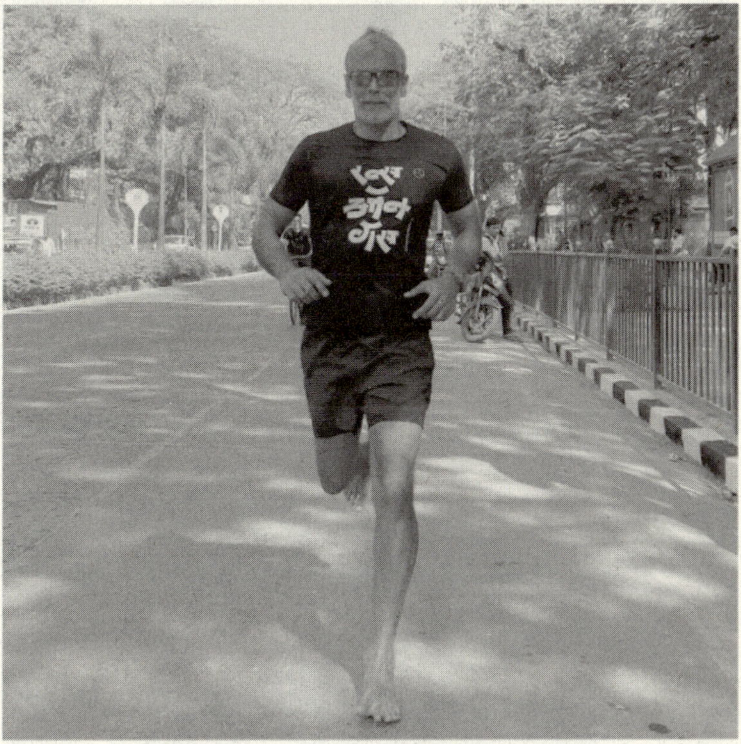

When Milind first started running barefoot, he found it difficult but soon began to enjoy it.

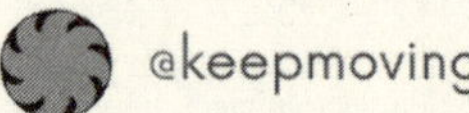

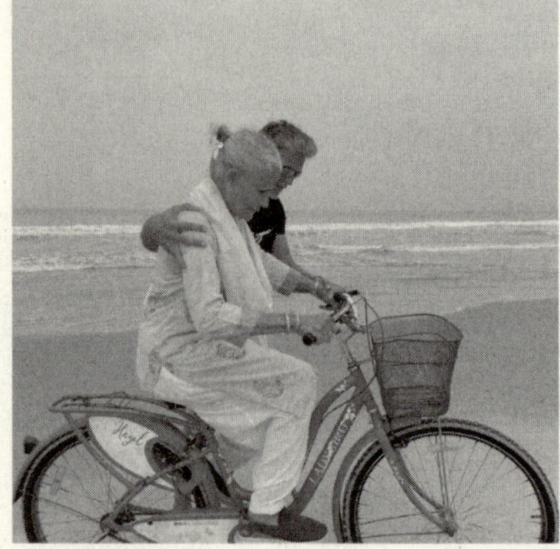

Usha cycling after 25 years!

@keepmoving

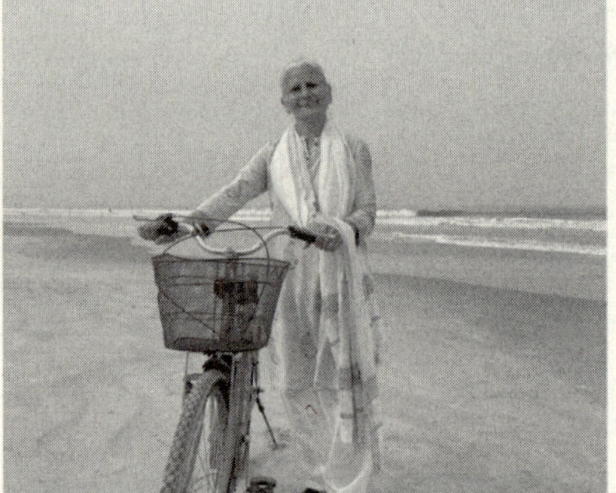

Usha's mantra: Never let anyone tell you that you are too old to do something.

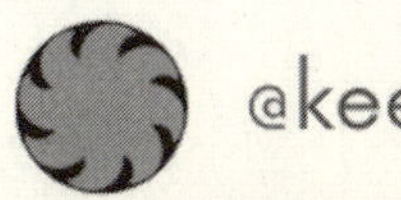 @keepmoving 

 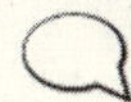 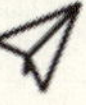 

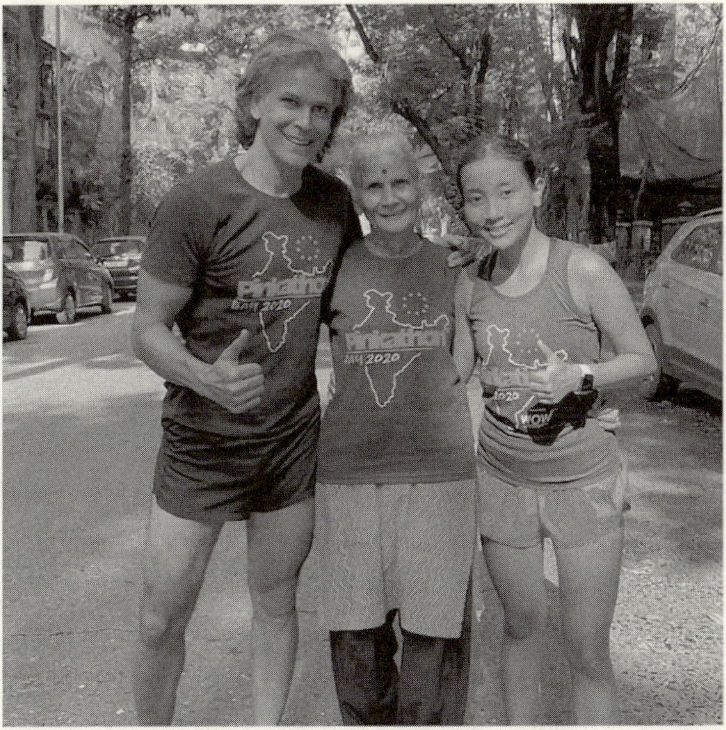

Pinkathon was founded in 2012 to inspire Indian women to get moving.

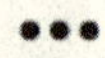

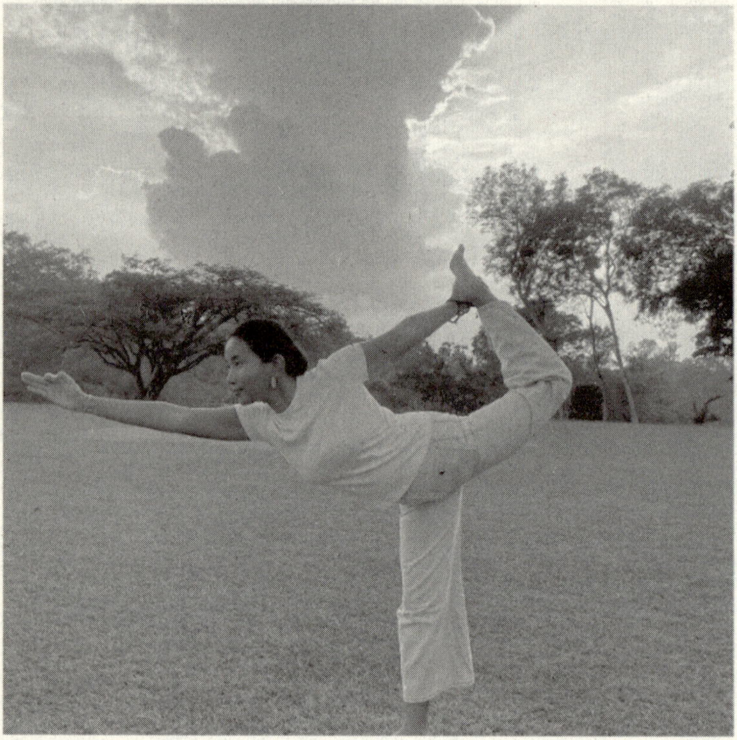

 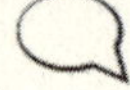  

Today Ankita is a certified yoga teacher.

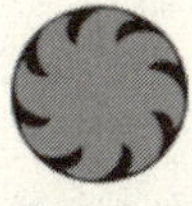

@keepmoving

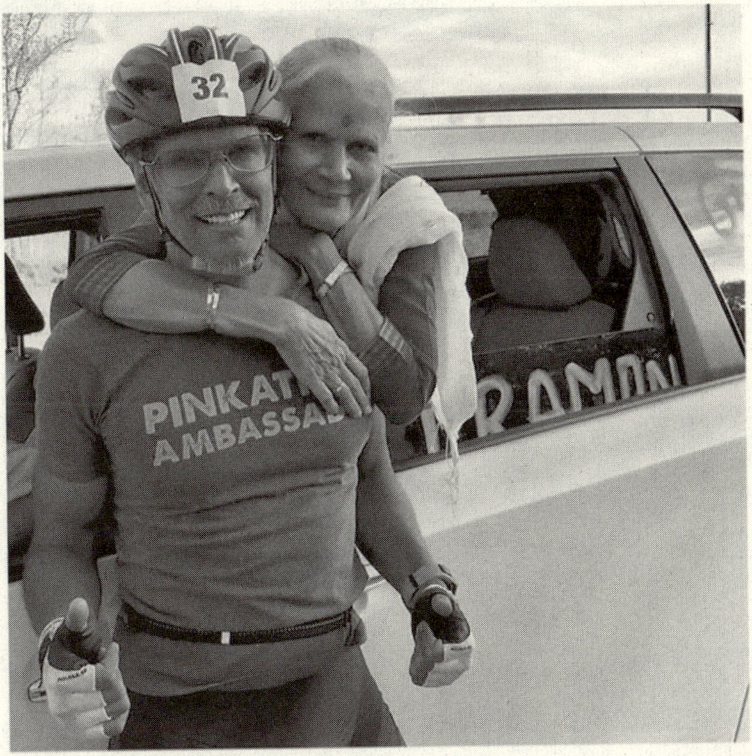

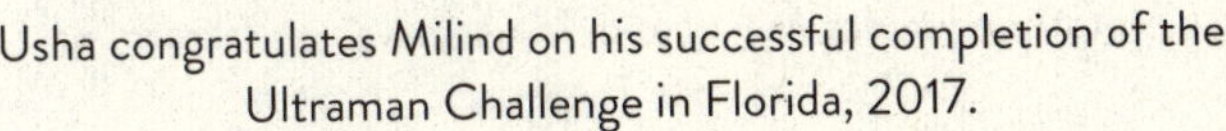

Usha congratulates Milind on his successful completion of the Ultraman Challenge in Florida, 2017.

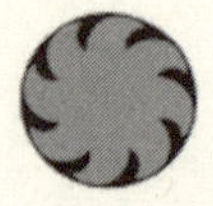 @keepmoving

  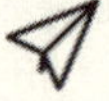 

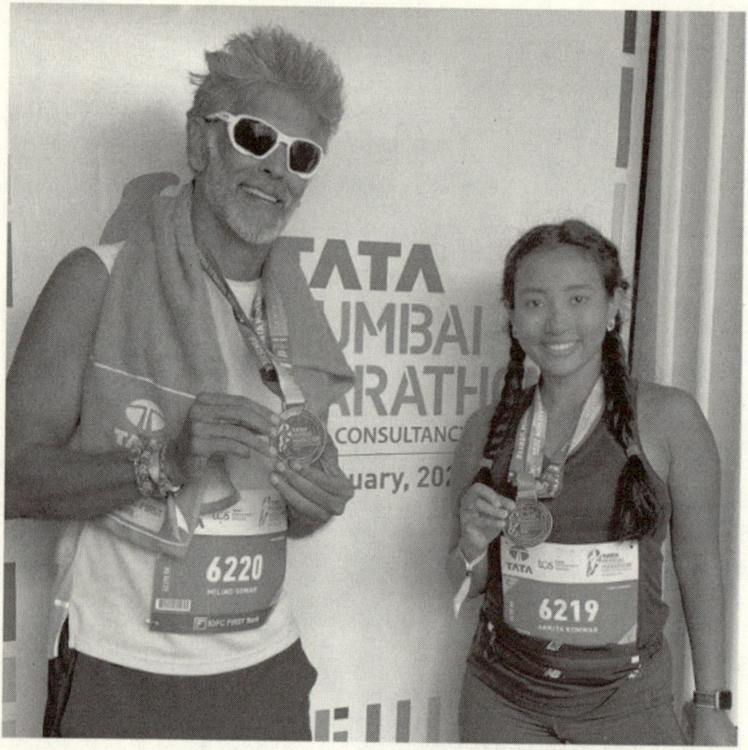

Marathon junkies Milind and Ankita have run marathons all over the world.

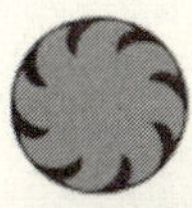

@keepmoving

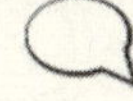

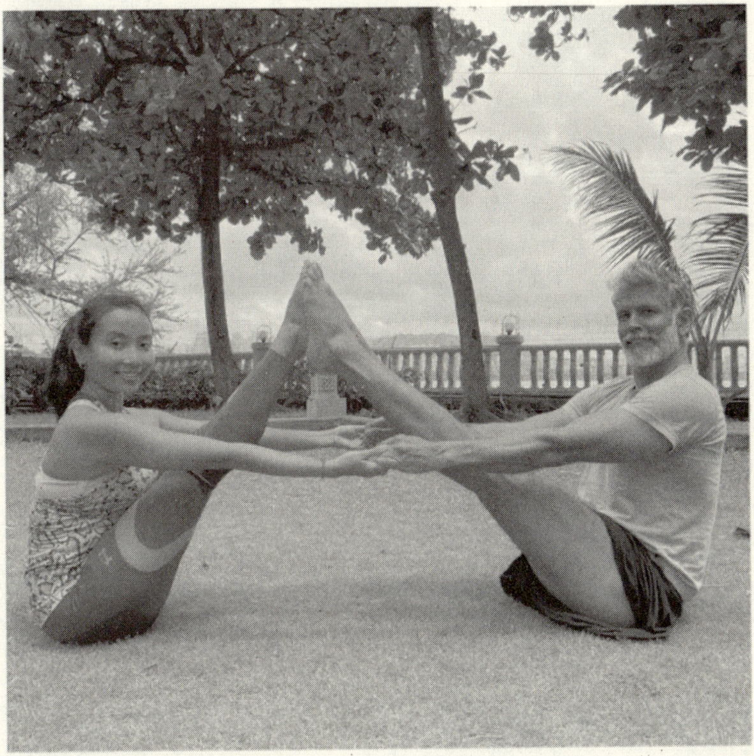

Couple goals!

A NOTE ON THE AUTHORS

Milind Soman, 58, is an actor, model, TV presenter and fitness evangelist. He has launched several initiatives, including Pinkathon, India's biggest women's run, to promote women's fitness and breast cancer awareness.

Ankita Konwar is a 32-year-old yoga practitioner and teacher. She has also completed several marathons and other feats of endurance.

Usha Soman is an 84-year-old retired biochemistry lecturer who has successfully completed numerous fitness challenges, including the 52 kilometre Sandakphu–Phalut winter trek, which she undertook at the age of 81.

Roopa Pai is the acclaimed writer of a number of books for adults and children including *The Gita for Children* and Milind Soman's memoir *Made in India*.